PROFOUND RETARDATION AND MULTIPLE IMPAIRMENT

Volume 2: Education and Therapy

PROFOUND RETARDATION AND MULTIPLE IMPAIRMENT

Volume 1: Development and Learning
Volume 2: Education and Therapy

Profound Retardation and Multiple Impairment

Volume 2: Education and Therapy

JAMES HOGG, Ph.D. and JUDY SEBBA, Ph.D,
Hester Adrian Research Centre, University of Manchester

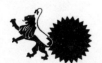

AN ASPEN PUBLICATION
Aspen Publishers, Inc.
Rockville, Maryland
1987

Library of Congress Cataloging in Publication Data

Hogg, J. (James)
    Profound Retardation and Multiple Impairment

    An Aspen Publication.
    Contents: V. 1. Development and Learning — V. 2.
Education and Therapy.
    Includes Index.
    1. Mentally Handicapped — Diseases. 2. Vision Disorders
3. Hearing Disorders. 4. Physically Handicapped.
5. Developmental Psychobiology. 6. Handicapped — Functional
Assessment. 7. Mentally Handicapped — Education. I. Sebba,
Judy. II. Title. (DNLM: 1. Handicapped. 2. Mental
Retardation. WM 300 H716P)
RC570.7.H64   1986   371.92'8   86-20670

Library of Congress Catalog Card Number: 86-20670
ISBN: 0-87189-310-X

CONTENTS

To our Parents
for their support and interest
over the years

PREFACE

In Volume 1 of this series, entitled *Development and Learning,* we presented a range of background material that we argued was essential if we are to understand the nature of profound retardation and multiple impairment. This material ranged from a general account of development and the effect of specific impairments on vision, hearing and physical development to a consideration of the nature of development and learning in people with profound retardation and multiple impairments. The value of the background presented in Volume 1 ultimately depends on how far it enables those working with this group of people to enhance development and adaptive functioning through intervention. In the present volume, we consider the other streams that must also be channelled into this activity.

In the opening chapter, we go beyond developmental assessment to consider a range of other instruments that contribute to the development of suitable programmes. These include measures of adaptive functioning as well as sensory and physical abilities. In Chapter 2, the elements of assessment are brought together in a wider account of a curriculum model that provides the overall framework for intervention with both children and adults. Succeeding chapters then deal with broad areas of the curriculum, notably, the development of cognition (Chapter 3), of communication (Chapter 4), of motor development and competence (Chapter 5) and of self-help skills (Chapter 6). In these chapters, much of the intervention work described draws heavily on the developmental background presented in Volume 1. In Chapter 7 we discuss behaviour problems in this population, and some of the main techniques that have been employed in dealing with them. Specifically we focus on self-injurious and stereotyped behaviour, though the techniques described are generalisable to other forms of behaviour disorder.

While much of the material we have drawn on is concerned with behavioural methods, we also offer accounts and where possible studies of other forms of therapy and intervention relevant to this group. In some instances, for example, physiotherapy, the main responsibility for such work will rest with a qualified professional. However, these activities cannot be exclusively restricted to such professionals, and we provide some background on the possible roles of teachers and trainers in these areas.

In order to ensure that these volumes were ever completed, some decisions had to be taken on what to omit from them. In the Preface to Volume 1 we commented that issues of care are not the whole story with respect to this group. While this is certainly the case, care activities and medical provision are essential elements in any service for people with profound retardation and multiple impairments. Issues of health care, use of drugs, control of epilepsy and so on have all been omitted. We hope to remedy this situation in a third, edited, volume to which specialists will contribute accessible accounts on a range of relevant issues. Similarly, we virtually excluded reference to the family needs of those with a son or daughter with profound retardation and multiple impairment. At present we are engaged in an extensive survey on this issue and hope that in due course this will be made available to the interested reader.

People with profound retardation and multiple impairments are unfathomable, in the sense that it is only with extreme difficulty that we can understand what they experience and their capacity for relating to and influencing the world around them. It is our hope that these volumes, whatever their imperfections, will focus attention on this group of people; that they will encourage those working in the field to acknowledge the complexity of their task and the extent of the information they are obliged to draw on if they are to fulfil this task effectively. We hope, too, that the books will stimulate more systematic studies of the understanding and abilities of people with profound retardation and multiple impairments, in order that the task of fathoming the unfathomable can be realised.

ACKNOWLEDGEMENTS

We would like to thank several people for their detailed reading of individual chapters in this volume, particularly Judith Coupe, Alison Frankenberg, Chris Kiernan, Elena Lieven, Peter Mittler, Ivan Tucker and David Wood. The chapters are undoubtedly improved as a result of their constructive and critical comments, though the shortcomings remain the writers' responsibility.

We are also grateful to those who have allowed us to use their assessment and curriculum material, notably Judy Bell, Christine Gunstone, Rebecca Fewell, John Presland, Gerry Simon, Jenny Warner and Chris Williams.

Many ideas have been derived from comments and discussions from participants and tutors involved in BIMH Workshops on 'The Education of People with Profound and Multiple Handicap', and from Colin Robson who has been engaged in evaluating this course.

Thanks, too, must be given to those people with whom we have worked over the years who are profoundly retarded and multiply handicapped and to their parents. It is encounters with them that have challenged our ideas and raised new questions to be addressed.

We are particularly indebted to Christine Houghton and Nicky Stoddart for typing the full manuscript of this volume and dealing with our continual and often disorganised requests for further changes.

Finally, we would like to express our gratitude to our families for their support over the years in which we have written these volumes.

1 BEYOND DEVELOPMENTAL ASSESSMENT

Introduction

In Volume 1 we demonstrated how children with profound retardation and multiple impairments could be considered in a framework of child development. In Chapter 7 of Volume 1 we reviewed some of the assessment procedures relevant to evaluating the cognitive status of such children in the sensorimotor and preoperational periods. Earlier, however, we described the high incidence of additional impairments in these children, and this state of affairs clearly has important consequences that take us beyond 'simple' psychological assessment.

The presence and influence of sensory of physical impairments suggests the need for an interdisciplinary approach to assessments, involving specialists such as physiotherapists, occupational therapists, audiologists, speech therapists, ophthalmologists and orthoptists. These specialists can provide detailed information with the implicated programme of management to minimise the development of additional impairments. However, an interdisciplinary approach should also include those people most closely involved with the handicapped person on a daily basis — the parents, teachers, instructors, nurses or residential staff. These people require assessment procedures which enable them continually to review their client's behaviour on a day to day basis and thereby modify or extend the daily programmes of intervention.

Our emphasis on 'interdisciplinary' rather than 'multidisciplinary' assessment reflects the authors' commitment to interactive assessment. This involves communication between the assessors rather than each professional separately observing the person and contributing their own written summary to the person's file. This chapter will consider the components of such an interdisciplinary assessment for children or adults with profound and multiple impairments, reviewing available procedures for assessing physical development, hearing, communication and prespeech skills and vision. However, further consideration will first be given to global assessments which attempt to cover many of these areas of development.

Psychometric Assessment

In Volume 1, Chapter 7 psychometric assessments were discussed. These procedures can be considered 'normative' in that they relate to normal developmental stages and usually yield an IQ score or developmental quotient. We have discussed how these assessments can provide information on the rate of development of children with multiple impairments and enable comparisons to be drawn between them and children whose development is normal. However, a number of limitations of using such procedures were pointed out, and further problems for assessment of children with profound and multiple impairments have emerged.

Global psychometric assessments which produce an overall score as an indicator of general ability may be misleading with a child whose severe sensory or physical impairments depress the total score relative to his or her score in each area of development outside the impaired modality. Moreover, as noted in Volume 1, Chapter 7, the inflexible nature of the procedures in many of these assessments, debars the use of alternative materials which might elicit the required response. Some tests start at beyond the 2 year old developmental level which limits their applicability to people with profound retardation, many of whom will be functioning below this level. Most are restricted to use by qualified testers, who, being strangers to the individual, may elicit atypical responses.

However, the primary disadvantage with psychometric procedures is that they do not indicate clearly which skills the person can and cannot do and do not therefore assist in the development of individual programme plans. These assessments are therefore primarily of use to administrators and researchers rather than to those working with the client on a daily basis. There has been a shift in recent years from assessment by the psychiatrist or psychologist to assessment by the teacher, nurse, parent or residential staff. This process has been accompanied by a move from using psychometric assessments to using criterion-referenced assessments, such as checklists which are not always related to a particular theory of child development but list specific skills in each area.

Criterion-Referenced Assessment

The distinction between psychometric procedures and criterion-referenced assessments is less clear than is sometimes suggested. Many checklists present skills in hierarchical order based on 'normal' development and are therefore 'normative'. Difficulties may arise from some checklists presenting skills in normative hierarchies and others not doing so, as the latter might be wrongly interpreted as hierarchically ordered, resulting in inappropriate choices of teaching targets. Furthermore, some psychometric procedures do include sections in which skills are listed which are scored according to the tester's observations of the person or the parents' or teacher's report of the person's behaviour. This procedure is the essence of what is involved in the completion of most checklists. A further source of confusion between the two approaches to assessment concerns the use of scores. Some checklists do provide scores attributing an identical score to each item on the list even though the items do not necessarily represent an equal step in development. It is perhaps this blurring of the distinctions between developmental and criterion-referenced assessments which has led to DuBose (1977) suggesting that combining these approaches might be beneficial as it might result in a curriculum in which skills are sequenced from easy to difficult and each tied to a daily living skill.

In varying degrees checklists have other limitations. For example, many do not cover all the areas of the curriculum required. The size of the steps between the items are often too large for people with profound retardation and multiple impairments, and in many checklists, there are not enough items that are relevant to individuals with such limited skills. The organisation of the skills on the checklist do not always assist teaching and record-keeping and as we shall consider in the next chapter, they are rarely written as clear objectives specifying conditions and criteria. This raises the question to be considered in Chapter 2, of how far the assessment should provide a basis for the curriculum. The specific checklists reviewed below can be evaluated against the disadvantages noted.

Checklists do, however, also have many advantages, the most important of which is probably their availability. They deal with important skill areas providing a structure or framework for keeping cumulative records. This can then provide a basis for discussion of the client's progress with parents and other professionals. They can be, and are, used by almost anybody. The Portage checklist (Shearer, Billingsley, Frohman, Hilliard, Johnson and Shearer 1972), for example, has been specifically designed to enable volunteers or professionals from any discipline to use it following a short period of training. Furthermore, checklists tend to be cheaper and more portable than other types of assessments.

There are many checklists available but only a few are applicable to people with profound retardation. Those reviewed here are the most widely used ones and those explicitly aimed at people with profound or multiple impairments. Initially, we will discuss general checklists which attempt to cover all the areas of development. Then, as we consider each component of the interdisciplinary assessment, we shall review any checklists addressing a specific area of development.

Two of the most widely used checklists in schools for children with severe learning difficulties, Social Education Centres and residential facilities have been the Adaptive Behavior Scale (ABS; Nihira, Foster, Shellhaas and Leland 1974) and the Progress Assessment Chart (PAC; Gunzburg 1963). The ABS is comprehensive and aimed at all ability levels but is rather long and therefore time-consuming with an unnecessary complex scoring system. One of its advantages to many staff is that it is one of the few criterion-referenced procedures applicable to adults with retardation although not specifically those who are profoundly retarded. Other scales not specifically aimed at children or those with profound retardation are the Developmental Checklist (Perkins, Taylor and Capie 1976) which provides a wide coverage of areas but not much detail within each area, and the Prescriptive Behavioral Checklists (Popovich 1977, 1981; Popovich and Laham 1981) which provide both wide coverage and almost too much detail.

Procedures devised originally for preschool children with developmental delay but which have been applied to children with profound retardation and even adults, are the Parental Involvement Project (PIP) charts (Jeffree and McConkey 1976), the Portage checklist (Shearer *et al.* 1972) and the Anson House Preschool Project Classroom Checklist (Gunstone 1979, revised 1985), illustrated in Figure 1.1. These checklists are clear and easy to follow, and perhaps for these reasons seem to be widely used but except for the latter one, have a paucity of items relevant to people with the most profound retardation. Other criterion-referenced assessments such as the PAC and the Social Training Achievement Record (Williams 1982a) illustrated in Figure 1.2 have attempted to present the information in a visual form and in the latter case in software form, perhaps to encourage staff to use them, but again, especially in relation to the PAC, have a lack of items applicable to those with profound retardation.

Turning to criterion-referenced assessments designed specifically for the child or adult with profound retardation, we should note examples such as the Behaviour Assessment Battery (BAB; Kiernan and Jones 1982) and the Bereweeke checklist (Mansell, Felce, Jenkins and Flight 1984). The BAB covers a wide range of the usual priority areas of self-help, postural and communication skills, but also includes visual and auditory behaviour, arguably more relevant in the assessment of the child

Figure 1.1: A Section of the Anson House Revised Checklist

	Sep	Oct	Nov	Dec	Jan	Feb	Mar	Apr	May	Jun	Jul
PRONE (Lying face down) 1. Head droops when suspended in prone: hand under tummy											
2. Head turns to side when child is placed on flat surface											
3. (a) Head lifted momentarily in mid line											
(b) Head turned to the side and lifted											
4. Head bobs up and down											
5. Takes weight on forearms - (a) Lift head up (May roll over to one side)											
(b) Lifts head up											
6. Makes swimming movements and pivots on floor (head up, legs and arms stretched)											
7. "Belly crawls" along floor using arms and legs (a) no pattern											
(b) in cross pattern											
8. Rolls from back to front											
9. Takes weight on hands and reaches for toys with support on one forearm											
10. Holds head well lifted, takes weight on abdomen and hands (pushes up: tummy on floor)											
11. Lifts one arm to reach for toy with other arm straight											
12. Pivots around to either side											
13. Gets on his/her tummy easily from sitting position											
14. Lifts head and chest while prone (Press up position - legs straight)											
15. Gets on hands and knees from prone and rocks											
16. Whilst on hands and knees reaches with hand for toy											

Source: Gunstone (1979, revised 1985 p. 2).

Figure 1.2: The Summary Scoring Sheet of the Social Training Achievement Record (STAR) Profile

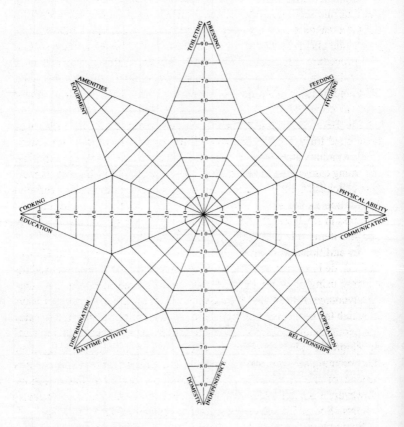

THE STAR PROFILE
Social Training Achievement Record

SUMMARY

Name_____Unit_____

Source: Williams, C. (1982a) *The Star Profile: Social Training Achievement Record,* British Institute of Mental Handicap, Kidderminster. Reproduced by kind permission of the publishers BIMH Publications.

with multiple impairments. This procedure has the advantage of focusing mainly on behaviours which are relevant because, for example, they are prerequisite skills to a vital behaviour such as 'weight-bearing' is for 'walking'. Furthermore, it covers sufficiently detailed behaviour to inform programme development by providing small steps between behaviours presented in lattices as in the example in Figure 1.3, although this leads to the disadvantage that the whole procedure is rather long to administer. The authors counterbalance this disadvantage by pointing out that one section can be selected once a decision has been made to devise a teaching programme in that particular area. The BAB attempts to include only behaviours which can be taught although it suggests that the procedure provides a basis for further analysis rather than a curriculum in itself. It provides an assessment applicable to those with profound handicaps but its use has perhaps been limited by the time it takes to complete.

The Bereweeke Skill Teaching System (Mansell *et al.* 1984) was developed for use in residential facilities by staff working with a wide range of adults and children. It includes a checklist, teaching activities, recording cards and other items and is described in full in the next chapter. The checklist is highly relevant to even those with the most profound retardation as the items start at a very early level of functioning and progress in small steps. The criteria for scoring are specified very clearly and the items relate directly to daily living skills.

An additional version of the checklist has been developed (Felce, Jenkins, de Kock and Mansell 1986) to make items more relevant to adults by only using adult-related materials as illustrated in Figure 1.4. One disadvantage of the Bereweeke System is that it does not suggest ways in which the procedures or criteria for scoring might be adapted to cater for people with additional impairments of vision, hearing or physical development. The section of the checklist on communication is rather disappointing as it is based on outdated and rigid behavioural procedures instead of the assessment of the functional use of communication. However, it is a highly applicable and easily used checklist for hospitals, schools, Social Education Centres and residential facilities alike.

Some checklists have been devised specifically for people with profound retardation and additional handicaps. *The Next Step on the Ladder* (Simon 1981) is an assessment and management guide for parents and professionals. It covers sight and hearing, movement, manual dexterity, social development, self-help skills and communication, this last section including both verbal and nonverbal items as illustrated in Figure 1.5. Each section begins with a checklist of relevant behaviours and is

Figure 1.3: Example of a Lattice and Some of the Corresponding Test Items from the Behaviour Assessment Battery

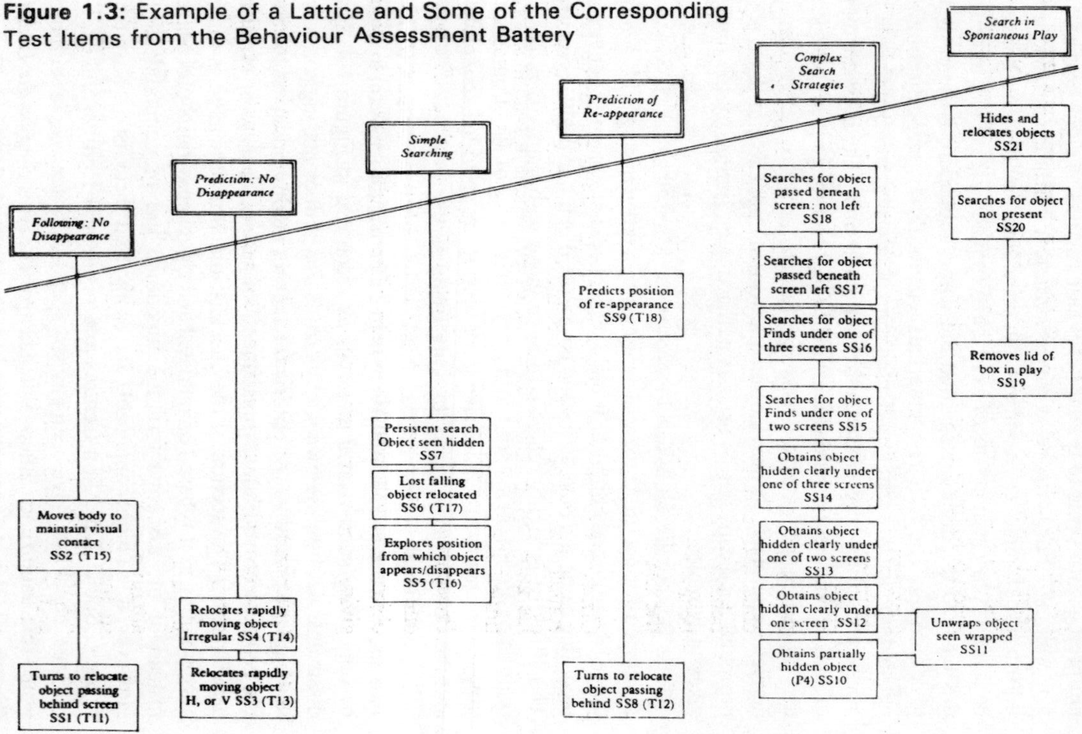

SS7   *Criterion Behaviour* — When the child has seen an object hidden under two screens he still searches for and obtains the object.

Presentation — The object is put under a half ball cover. A second screen, an orange cloth, is then laid over the ball. The child is not allowed to begin searching for the object for three seconds following the completion of the procedure.

SS8   *Criterion Behaviour* — The child looks at an object and follows
(T12)   its movements along a trajectory which passes behind him. The child then turns his head to relocate the object as it reappears.

Presentation — The object should be presented at the side of the child and his attention drawn to it. The object is slowly moved behind the child to reappear to him on his other side. This behaviour may also be seen if examiner walks quietly behind the child.

SS9   *Criterion Behaviour* — When an object which is moving hori-
(T18)   zontally passes out of sight behind a screen, the child will shift his gaze to the point where the object would appear if it continued along its original path.

Presentation — The object is shown to the child about 20 cms to one side of the screen. When the child is looking move the object slowly behind the screen. Care should be taken to avoid giving cues by arm movements.

SS10   *Criterion Behaviour* — When an object is partially hidden beneath
(P4)   a screen within easy grasping distance of the child, the child obtains the object.

Presentation — The object is put on the table and the child's attention drawn to it. The half ball is then put over the object so that it partially covers it. A delay of about three seconds is imposed between the completion of the presentation procedure and encouraging or allowing the child to respond.

SS11   *Criterion Behaviour* — The child unwraps a cloth that was folded round an object whilst he was watching. He ignores the cloth once it has been removed.

Source: Kiernan and Jones (1982 pp. 99 and 167).

Figure 1.4: A Section from the Bereweeke Checklist for Adults

COGNITIVE

Item	Materials/Procedures	Performance	Assessment	Remarks
1. Copies gesture	Wave at client. Say 'Do this'	Waves back	☐	
2. Copies simple action	2 mugs. Put 1 mug in open cupboard. Ask client to copy	Puts mug in cupboard	☐	
3. Matches object	2 identical tins/jars/packets. Put 1 of each pair in cupboard reasonably apart, door left open. Put other of each pair on work surface in non-corresponding order. (Can be assessed naturally after shopping)	Puts tin next to tin, jar next to jar, packet next to packet	☐	
4. Matches objects by picture/label	3 pairs of tins all same size with distinctively different labels. Put 1 of each pair in cupboard reasonably apart, door left open. Put other of each pair on work surface in non-corresponding order	Puts tins with same label together	☐	

#	Skill	Instruction	Criterion	
5.	Points to objects which are the same	4 pots of jam, 2 the same. Ask 'Which pots are the same?'	Points to the 2 which are the same	☐
6.	Copies complex action	Cutlery and mats for 2 place settings. Lay 1 setting. Ask client to copy	Lays place setting as shown	☐
7.	Matches objects to picture/label	3 labels from tins/jars. Go shopping. Ask client to get 1 tin/jar for each label	Gets objects to match	☐
8.	Sorts by shape	Number of knives, forks and spoons	Sorts cutlery into knife, fork and spoon groups	☐
9.	Sorts by colour	Pile of different coloured clothes/towels	Sorts into piles according to colour	☐
10.	Sorts by size	Number of serving, dessert and tea spoons	Sorts cutlery into separate groups	☐
11.	Copies speech	Say 'Goodbye' to client	Says 'Goodbye'	☐

Source: Felce et al. (1986, p.15).

Figure 1.5: A Section of *The Next Step on the Ladder* Checklist

---

Developmental assessment

A | **RECEPTIVE**

VERBAL: UNDERSTANDING SPEECH AND SOUND

NOTE.   This section is appropriate for the child who can hear adequately.

The first four steps below are similar to items 1-4 in Section I. Use of sight and hearing (page 23/24). Steps 5-12 are designed to advance the use of hearing which is known to be there.

1	Shows startle response to sudden loud noise when source of sound is not visible.
2	Becomes still momentarily after sound is made when source is not visible.
*3	Turns or moves head/eyes towards sound.
4	Quietens at sound of soothing voice, becomes distressed by sharp, "angry" tones.
*5	Reaches out towards objects when sounds are made with them.
*6	Locates and turns towards sounds coming from a greater distance or when sound source is above or below ear level.
7	Responds to "No" by stopping current activity.
8	Turns to own name and begins to learn the meaning of simple verbal instructions.
9	Differentiates between two or more sound-making objects.
10	Differentiates objects by their names.
11	Points to three or more body parts on request.
12	Follows more complex instructions.

*Some blind children have increased difficulty in locating sounds and, for them, Items 3, 5 and 6 may be achieved later than items 4 and 7.

NON VERBAL: UNDERSTANDING SIGNS AND GESTURE

NOTE.   This section is appropriate for the child with limited hearing but sufficient vision to appreciate what is happening.

1	Shows awareness when touched.
2	Tries to locate adult by reaching when touched.
*3	Watches adult actions.
4	Anticipates and carries out simple actions.
5	Anticipates routine activity.
6	Understands the meaning of familiar objects and actions.
7	Carries out familiar actions when prompted by simple signs.
*8	Understands one or two standard signs.
*9	Understands three or more standard signs.

*Item 3 will not apply if the child is totally blind. In items 8 and 9 the signs used must involve an actual touch (see illustrations of "natural" signs, page 135).

Source: Simon, G.B. (1981) *The Next Step on the Ladder,* British Institute of Mental Handicap, Kidderminster, p. 109. Reproduced by kind permission of the publishers BIMH Publications.

followed by suggested activities. These activities are illustrated by drawings and the approach appears to have been well received by those working with children with multiple impairments although staff working with adults are less comfortable with the drawings depicting children. We shall further consider this procedure in relation to models of curriculum development in Chapter 2.

The assessment manual produced by Collins and Rudolph (1975) for deaf-blind multi-handicapped children covers the same areas as *The Next Step on the Ladder* with an additional section on cognition covering object-related behaviour, memory, matching, classification, etc.. This manual is very detailed and like the Popovich and Anson House checklists, lengthier than most of the others reviewed here. However, this detail makes it very relevant to the child with profound retardation since it has, for example, twelve items on head control alone. Furthermore, there is an extensive list of items on signing and prespeech skills which are still omitted in many more recently developed checklists.

The reasons for the growing popularity of these criterion-referenced assessments is emphasised by DuBose and Langley (1977) whose own Developmental Activities Screening Inventory, like many of the procedures described above, is aimed at people in daily contact with the person — teachers, nurses, parents or residential staff. They point out that these informal assessments encourage observation of the person in the situation most conducive to the use of the particular skill being considered. Checklists enable staff or parents to observe, for example, self-help skills while the person is eating and using the toilet, language skills during non-directed play and even less obviously related naturalistic observation such as motor skills during dressing. DuBose and Langley's finding that their Inventory with its adaptation for visually impaired and non-communicating children correlates with more formal normative-referenced measures further illustrates the usefulness of criterion-referenced approaches. Their use has been extended by staff devising their own checklists with items relating specifically to their clients and the particular setting in which they work.

The Assessment of Physical Impairment

The importance of involving a physiotherapist in the interdisciplinary assessment of the person with multiple impairments as early as possible cannot be overemphasised. There are two main reasons for this: the need to limit the effects of impairment and the identification of realistic limitations on physical development, which the nonspecialist may have overlooked. These will be considered in turn before describing the main approaches to assessment of physical skills. Finally, procedures designed to be used by nonphysiotherapists will be reviewed.

Limiting the Effect of Impairment

Identification as early as possible of the correct methods of handling and positioning the child to arrest the development of abnormal postural reflexes or muscle tone is crucial. Correct positioning reduces the likelihood of auditory and visual perception remaining under-developed due to the presence of physical impairments (see Volume 1, Chapter 6). Any possibility that the success of educational programmes could be undermined by incorrect handling or positioning must be reduced.

Detailed physiotherapy assessments include detection of joint stiffness which can lead to the prevention of joint contractures and muscle weakness for which steps can be taken to prevent the formation of deformities due to muscle imbalance. Furthermore, any persistence of normal postural reflexes beyond the stage at which they usually disappear may inhibit the child's development. If postural reflexes gain in strength and dominate the child's motor activity they can prevent further motor development. For example, the persistence of the Asymmetrical Tonic Neck Reflex beyond 4 months makes rolling over difficult or impossible, prevents the child from getting his or her hands together in the midline and inhibits self-feeding and ambulation. Identification of abnormal reflex reactions is therefore crucial in the limiting of the effects of the impairment.

The Identification of Realistic Limitations on Physical Developments

In Volume 1, Chapter 3 (pp. 64–6 and 75–82), we described Touwen's approach to assessment and development of fine and gross motor skills as an aid to neurological assessment. We have seen above how persistence of one abnormal pattern of movement can inhibit the development of other physical skills. If neuromuscular restrictions are too great there may be limitations on the development of some physical skills even when thorough assessment by a physiotherapist has led to correct handling, positioning and appropriate use of aids. Unlimited appropriate application of behavioural or other teaching techniques cannot achieve a skill in a person whose neuromuscular limitations prevent that skill from developing. Detailed physiotherapy assessment leading to the identification of realistic limitations for each person is therefore essential to ensure we do not undermine the confidence or time of client, parents or staff by struggling to teach inappropriate physical skills.

Assessment Procedures Used by Physiotherapists

Commonly used assessment procedures for physiotherapists include the assessment of general physical ability, range of joint movement, muscle strength and reflex reactions. These procedures are described by Holt (1965) and Levitt (1982) and their application to a group of children with profound retardation and multiple impairments is described in detail in Sebba (1978). Levitt emphasises the need to select assessment methods that link directly to the techniques of treatment.

Physical Ability Chart

The Physical Ability Charts described by Holt (1965) and Levitt (1982) include a list of functional gross motor skills in the order of normal development with approximate age norms for each item given ranging from 1 week to 3 years. The items are scored on a rating scale ranging from 'no ability' to 'normal performance'. This provides a record of individual gross motor skills and identifies the stages reached by the person in prone, supine and upright development. It also supplies a method of estimating the next steps of development and the possibility of foreseeing the likely blocking factors in the achievement of that step. If used as an ongoing method of assessment, by repeating observations regularly, this procedure could be used to evaluate the person's progress both on isolated motor skills and on general prone, supine and upright development.

There are two disadvantages with the Physical Ability Chart. The first concerns the use of the rating scales involved which depend on the subjective judgement of the observer. This may be more problematic for the middle ratings than for those at either end concerned with the total absence of a skill or normal performance. The use of more than one observer may enable reliability of the scale to be established. The second disadvantage is that the chart does not include either fine motor functioning or self-help skills both of which are covered by other assessments described in this chapter. As previously suggested, it is quite possible to observe many skills during daily living activities and gross motor skills lend themselves particularly well to this approach.

Assessment of the Range of Joint Movement

The range of all possible movements in each of the joints of the limbs, neck and the spinal column is assessed. Shoulder movements may be measured with the shoulder blade fixed and free in order to detect the exact location of the stiffness. The position of adjacent joints is stated where appropriate. Some muscles reach over two joints and tightness can only be detected by extending the muscle in both joints. On the rating sheet, the normal range is given for comparative purposes. Each joint movement is scored as full, stiff or limited and right or left sides and passive or active movements are indicated where appropriate.

Assessment of Muscle Strength

The assessment of muscle strength described by Holt (1965) is based on the work of Bobath and Bobath (1956). The strength of individual muscle groups is measured since each possible movement is affected by a group of muscles. The scoring is done on a rating scale from complete paralysis to contraction against powerful resistance. This procedure is used to detect muscle weakness and thereby take steps to prevent the formation of deformities due to muscle imbalance. Molnar and Alexander (1983) refer to a variety of procedures aimed at providing objective measurement of muscle strength using equipment designed to isolate the movements.

There are two main disadvantages with applications of these muscle strength assessments to people with profound impairments. First, the procedures rely on the person's comprehension of commands and ability to isolate movements, both of these involving skills that tend to be lacking in this population. Many people with multiple impairments have muscles which work in total patterns such as total flexion or total extension. This may lead to an inability to differentiate, for example, between bending a knee and bending a whole leg.

Secondly, consideration of muscle strength may be less relevant to the assessment of physical development in some people with multiple impairments, since the person's movements are affected more by their cerebral palsy than by their muscle strength *per se*. Hence, the person's muscles may be quite strong but they may lack the ability to control them. For example, the extensor muscles are strong in the case of extensor spasticity in the legs but the flexors will be weak. The flexor strength cannot be measured or increased without first inhibiting the extensor spasm. The assessment of muscle strength may therefore be less important than that of muscle tone, abnormal movements and the presence or absence of reflex reactions.

The Assessment of Reflex Reactions

Examples of assessments of reflex reactions can be found in Holt (1965; 1975) and Levitt (1982). The person is positioned and moved in an attempt to evoke any abnormal postural reflexes that may be present. The absence of normal postural reflexes is also revealed. It should be noted that it is sometimes the persistence of a normal postural reflex beyond the age at which it usually disappears, which makes that reflex abnormal. For example, the Asymmetrical Tonic Neck Reflex is usually present at birth to 4 months, but its presence at 3 years would clearly be considered abnormal.

Assessment Procedures Used by Nonphysiotherapists

It is clear that assessment of physical development in people with multiple impairments is a complex problem. Hence, the need to involve a physiotherapist in the interdisciplinary assessment process is seen as essential. However, the physiotherapist is a scarce resource usually only available for any particular client on a once a week or once a fortnight basis. For this reason, many physiotherapists have interpreted their role as partly involved with the transfer of skills to parents and staff in daily contact with the client. If we regard continual assessment as a means of regularly evaluating individual programmes it may be useful for the person carrying out these programmes to have criterion-referenced assessments as a framework. All of the general criterion-referenced assessments described above include sections on gross and fine motor skills. Three procedures will be mentioned here, two of which (Presland 1982; Webb, Schultz and McMahill 1977) are aimed specifically at assessing motor skills in children and adults with profound and multiple impairments. The third (Hogg 1978) is aimed at assessing fine motor skills at all ability levels.

Paths to Mobility in 'Special Care' (Presland 1982) is a guide to checklist and teaching suggestions which will be further discussed in Chapter 2. The checklist covers development in lying, sitting, kneeling, crawling, standing and walking. Its particular appeal to work with people with profound retardation is the very small steps between items at the early stages of development illustrated in Figure 1.6 and by the 72 items it covers before even getting to the stage of sitting! The specific appeal it may have to those working with people with multiple impairments is that it has sections on walking with crutches, walking with sticks and using a wheelchair. While many of the items covered in the Physical Ability Chart used by physiotherapists are also mentioned in this checklist, the comprehensive detail given in the checklist, the wording of items as objectives and the linking-in with teaching suggestions, makes this a valuable tool for those concerned with daily programmes.

Figure 1.6: Sections of the *Paths to Mobility* Checklist

	Criteria	Date tested	Date mastered	Date checked

Section 4. ROLLING
1. On back, rolls part way to side.
2. On side, rotates head towards ceiling.
3. On side, rolls on to back.
4. On front, rolls part way to side.
5. On back, rolls to side.
6. On front, rolls head and chest, or legs and hips, to "on-back" position.
7. On back, rolls head and chest, or legs and hips, to side.
8. On front, rolls on to back.
9. On back, rolls head and chest, or legs and hips, to "on-front" position.
10. On back, rolls to front.
11. Moves around by rolling.

Section 5. HELD AGAINST SHOULDER
1. Holds head upright for 2 seconds or more.
2. Holds head upright for 10 seconds or more.
3. Swayed from side to side, holds head steady.
4. Swayed backwards and forwards, holds head steady.

Section 6. SITTING
1. Allows self to be placed in sitting position on adult lap.
2. Allows self to be placed in sitting position on surface.
3. Held in sitting position, holds head erect 2 seconds or more.
4. Held in sitting position, holds head erect continuously, but with "bobbing" movements.
5. Pulled from lying on back to sitting, lifts head in line with body towards end of movement.
6. Propped in sitting position, holds head steady for 10 minutes or more.
7. Propped in sitting position, maintains only a slight curve in the back for 10 minutes or more.
8. Pulled from lying on back to sitting, elbows, wrists, and fingers straighten (instead of bending as formerly).
9. Placed in sitting position with adult's hand supporting only lower part of back, maintains position 2 seconds or more.
10. Pulled from lying on back to sitting, lifts head in line with body before halfway to sitting position.

Source: Presland, J. (1982), *Paths to Mobility in 'Special Care'*, British Institute of Mental Handicap, Kidderminster, p. 54. Reproduced by kind permission of the publishers BIMH Publications.

The Glenwood Awareness, Manipulation and Posture (AMP) Scale (Webb *et al.* 1977) is designed to evaluate the sensorimotor functioning of children who are grossly handicapped. The Awareness scale covers avoidance, approach and integrating memory with present stimuli, but the Manipulation scale covers posture and mobility. Hence, although these scales are not exclusively on motor skills, a substantial part of them is relevant here. Each item is assessed through a more formal testing procedure than the naturalistic observation implied in the Presland checklist. Furthermore, the procedure involves an observer who presents the items to the person and should be familiar to him or her and an evaluator who records the response and should be a comparative stranger. Thus, the demands this procedure makes on personnel may limit its use in schools, adult day services, hospitals and other agencies.

The Fine Motor Skill Assessment Battery (Hogg 1978) was developed to enable assessment of young children with developmental delay regardless of the nature or degree of impairment. The items are organised into ten sections on postural control, visual function, reaching for objects, object insertion, placement of tubes, using a scoop, placement of flat objects, block stacking, bead threading and complex sub-assembly. The battery has items relevant to the child with profound retardation provided they are able to pick up an object, as illustrated in Figure 1.7.

The Assessment of Hearing

In Volume 1, Chapter 1 it was noted that people with profound retardation were more likely to have a hearing loss than those with less severe retardation. In fact we referred to studies suggesting that with increasing severity of mental retardation there is an increasing likelihood of sensory impairments. Early detection of hearing loss has become more probable with the introduction of routine hearing tests. In this section we will consider the rationale for early detection of hearing loss, the methods used by audiologists and other specialists to assess hearing and methods available for nonspecialists such as teachers, nurses, parents, etc.

The population focused on by this book is clearly at greater risk of having hearing losses. In Volume 1, Chapter 5 the developmental consequences of such impairments were considered in detail. It will suffice here to reiterate that normal auditory ability is a prerequisite to normal development of language and communication. While this area of development may remain limited in the clients with whom we are concerned, further restrictions arising from hearing problems can be avoided.

Figure 1.7: An Item from the Fine Motor Skill Assessment Battery

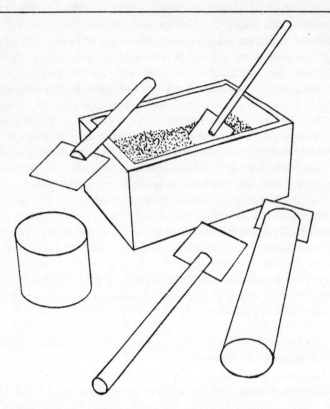

Place scoop and sandbox in front of child working from largest diameter scoop to smallest. Say 'Pick it up'. If necessary follow Indicative Sequence.

Target behaviour:

Child successfully scoops sand onto scoop and raises scoop from sandbox transferring sand to beaker. Record success/failure. Classify grip. Note any use of non-scoop hand. Record Indicative Sequence.

Source: Hogg (1978 p. 29).

Furthermore, as Williams (1982b) has indicated, some of the people who are labelled as having severe retardation may in fact have profound hearing losses which may be concealing their normal or near-normal intelligence.

The availability of equipment and methods of alleviating hearing losses suggest that thorough assessment is a worthwhile investment. In the Cunningham and McArthur (1981) study, described in Volume 1, Chapter 1, the hearing of half the Down's Syndrome infants tested improved following surgery or treatment with decongestants. There is no reason to suppose that middle ear problems such as these could not be treated successfully in people with profound retardation.

In Chapter 2, we shall be discussing the establishment of possible reinforcers as one aspect of teaching approaches. Assessing the extent of a hearing loss is important in relation to this as many readily available toys and pieces of equipment (such as the 'Pethna' toys (Woods and Parry 1981), microcomputer software, etc.) have built in reinforcers involving auditory feedback. If the person has a hearing loss but responds to raised levels of input, it is clearly worthwhile pursuing the presentation of stimuli through the auditory modality whereas profound deafness would suggest switching to other modalities. If other modalities are impaired, there may be more dependence on auditory cues, suggesting that any residual hearing must be assisted as much as possible.

One problem which arises in relation to people with profound and multiple impairments is establishing whether lack of responses to auditory stimuli are due to a hearing loss or in keeping with the general level of retardation. As we shall see, procedures have been developed to distinguish between these two. For management purposes it is important to establish which of these explanations is correct, since hearing aids or amplification may damage a person's ear if inappropriately used. Failing to use amplification when a hearing loss exists may seriously restrict the amount of auditory information received.

Assessments Used by Audiologists

The three assessment procedures described below are the distraction test, the impedance bridge measurement and electrical response audiometry. The first two of these are widely available and the distraction procedure is used in the local authority screening offered to all children. In addition to these three procedures an otological examination by an ear, nose and throat specialist may be carried out if this is suggested but a description of this is beyond the scope of this chapter.

The Distraction Procedure. The person is placed on their parent's lap with the back to the parent, or seated on a chair unassisted if able to sit unsupported. One tester stands directly in front of the person and distracts him or her by using toys, eye contact and vocalisations. A second tester stands slightly behind the person (out of her or his peripheral vision) to one side at a distance of three feet and presents an auditory stimulus on a level with the person's ear.

The timing of the presentation of the stimulus is crucial and is indicated by the first tester who stops distracting the person at this point. The intensity of the stimulus presented is increased until the person responds and the intensity at this point is measured by a Sound Level Meter. A response is usually a head turn and is regarded as consistent if shown twice to both low frequency and high frequency sounds on each side. Other responses such as eye blink, or eye movements, startle response and smiling are noted. All responses are reinforced using verbal, social and physical rewards.

The side on which the stimuli are presented is randomised in order to avoid position biases. Distraction by the first tester is continued during any movements of the second tester behind the person. The distraction is sometimes used without it being followed by a sound to reduce learned response patterns. Knowledge of previous testing of the person is obtained to avoid learned responses influencing results. Items used for sound production include rattles, chimebars, voice (but only from the larynx, i.e. not a whisper), the vowel 'oo' which is sometimes used as a low frequency stimulus, and warble tones from an audiometer. A voice shouting 'Ba' is used to elicit the auropalpebral reflex (eye blink to sound).

The distraction tests are used to elicit simple responses to sound and to measure the decibel level of the sounds at the moment the response is given. The tests establish differential responses to high and low frequency sounds which may be crucial since a loss in only one range of frequencies may distort sound reception rather than reducing it. Thus, any hearing loss discovered can be treated appropriately with respect to volume and frequency of sounds.

There are a number of problems which arise in the use of distraction tests for assessing people with multiple impairments. In infants with no impairments, the localisation of a sound source by head turning usually develops by about 4 months although eye movements to sound are present from birth (Bower 1974). However, if the person has poor head or trunk control as may occur in an individual with physical impairments, this response to sounds may not be elicited. Furthermore, poor motor control may make it difficult, if not impossible, to position the person suitably for the tests to be administered, so as to ensure the ears are not restricted.

The infant with visual impairments has been noted to develop head turning and eye movements in response to a sound in early infancy but this response usually disappears by 6 months of age (Freedman 1964). Bower (1974) has argued that since localisation of sound is present at birth it cannot be a learned response. It is perhaps not maintained because children learn that they gain no further information by head turning and are therefore not reinforced for this behaviour.

The person with a hearing loss might be expected to make frequent random visual checks by head turning in order to increase their visual field to compensate for the loss of auditory information. This visual checking may appear more rapidly in a person whose hearing loss is restricted to one ear only. Thus, the testers must be cautious in their interpretation of a lack of head-turning responses and must take procedural measures to establish consistency in people with frequent and rapid head-turning responses.

A further problem relates to the application of this procedure as a screening device used on a wider scale, usually by health visitors. When distraction procedures are used for screening, rather than diagnostically as described above, the procedure simply involves noting whether or not a head-turning response is given to minimal level high and low frequency sounds. Sound level meters are not therefore usually used and occasionally a child is tested with only one tester thereby negating the crucial aspect of this procedure i.e. the distractor. Furthermore, background noise levels during screening may invalidate the results.

Some of these reasons may have contributed to the questionable reliability of the local authority screening noted in the Cunningham and McArthur study in which 50 per cent of the infants passed this screening but consistently failed when tested by independent audiologists. There is little doubt that the person with multiple impairments is difficult to test and it has been suggested (Cunningham and McArthur 1981; Tucker and Nolan 1984) that all such individuals should be automatically referred to audiology clinics where greater experience is available. The distraction procedure alone cannot provide sufficient information to be conclusive about the hearing of people with multiple impairments. Assessing this population requires the audiologist to use information from all procedures conducted, to build up a picture of the individual's hearing.

The Impedance Bridge Measurement. The impedance bridge measurement involves fitting the person with an ear probe through which a pure sound is passed, resulting in alteration of the air pressure exerted on the drum. The amount of sound transmitted through the ear and the amount being returned is then measured and is illustrated by the tympanogram using an automatic recorder. Stapedial reflex thresholds can also be measured using this equipment. Any conductive hearing loss in the middle ear will be indicated by a flatter compliance curve than that which is derived from normal middle ear functioning.

The impedance bridge measurements are particularly useful if the distraction tests have failed to establish any consistent responses to sounds. The person's lack of responses on distraction tests may be attributed to attentional rather than hearing defects (Taylor 1968) but the lack of a hearing deficit must still be established. In difficult-to-test people, the impedance bridge measurement procedure is relatively simple to carry out and can indicate the presence of middle ear disorders, which can lead to the person being referred to an ear, nose and throat specialist.

Two major problems arise in relation to the impedance bridge measurement procedure. First, the finding that the compliance curves are normal still does not enable assurance that the stimulus is reaching the brain since there may be a sensorineural hearing loss. The procedure therefore still fails to inform the tester of whether a person with profound retardation has a sensorineural hearing loss or is just not responding due to general retardation. The answer to this can only really be established through use of electrical response audiometry described below.

The second problem of using impedance bridge measurements concerns the need for people to be in good health at the time of testing. Prolonged catarrhal problems and repeated infections lead to a flatter compliance curve which would indicate a conductive hearing loss. In this situation the results would be misleading since the hearing loss might only be temporary, with normal hearing resuming when the catarrh clears.

Electrical Response Audiometry. Electrical Response Audiometry (ERA) procedures and some of the limitations of assessing hearing using them are described more fully in Barratt (1980) and Tucker and Nolan (1984). They involve testing the functioning of parts of the neural hearing pathway and are particularly useful to determine hearing thresholds in people who are not amenable to testing by conventional methods. The physiological principle behind ERA is that when a nerve is activated it undergoes electrical changes. Electrodes are attached to the person's head so that the electrical activity of the brain can be recorded. A sound is then presented through the headphones and a computer samples the resulting activity of the nerves in the hearing system. The auditory evoked response is built up by repeating the sound and the response is visually displayed as a wave form on the screen of the computer.

There are four main types of electrical responses commonly used for hearing assessment; the electrocochleographic response, the brain stem electric response, the post-auricular muscle response and the slow vertex response. The brain stem electric response is particularly suitable for assessing the hearing of people with multiple impairments as the response is unaffected by drugs or whether the person is awake or asleep, thus enabling the person to be sedated if necessary. Both this response and the electrocochleographic response are very reliable but both only give measures of high frequency hearing. The slow vertex response gives information about hearing thresholds at all frequencies but is greatly affected by the arousal state of the person and drugs and requires prolonged attention to the sound stimuli. It is therefore less suitable for our target population. The post-auricular muscle response has been found to be less reliable (Barratt 1980).

The disadvantages of using electrical response audiometry with people with multiple impairments are mainly problems to do with using the procedures *per se* and the relative recency of their development. The equipment required is very expensive and not readily available. Highly trained and experienced testers are required to interpret the results accurately, and the results are easily affected by sources of interference such as muscular activity, electrical interference from machines or flourescent lights and neurological damage in the person which can produce abnormally shaped waveforms. Difficulties can arise when assessing lower frequency ranges but attempts to elicit responses to voice and other low frequency stimuli and the use of impedance bridge measurements, will again enable the audiologist to build up a picture of the individual's hearing. Electrical response procedures provide the only real method of detecting whether auditory stimulation is reaching the brain in a person with profound retardation and multiple impairments.

Assessment Procedures Used by Nonaudiologists

Screening infants for hearing losses is now an established routine service offered to most parents in most areas. However, many of the children and adults with multiple impairments with whom we are concerned here are unlikely to give any responses in the distraction procedure used for screening described above. Hence, these individuals will require audiological assessment using impedance bridge measurements and possibly electrical response audiometry. Unfortunately many of these individuals are beyond the age at which routine testing is offered and even for those who are likely to be tested the delay from referral to assessment can be long because of the tremendous backlog of 'difficult-to-test' clients. Furthermore, more information available to the audiologist from observations by those in closest contact with the individual can only provide a valuable contribution to the specialist's assessment. For these reasons, attempts to produce auditory assessments that can be used by nonaudiologists will be described.

The particular contribution that can be made by the nonspecialist to auditory assessment is information on the auditory behaviour of the person with multiple impairments across a variety of situations in their daily environment. Procedures reported for assessment of hearing by the nonspecialist have therefore been based on observational techniques rather than on any advanced technological equipment. Kershman and Napier (1982) describe how parents, teachers and teachers' aides were able to establish reliability on observations of behaviours shown by children with multiple impairments in response to a variety of auditory stimuli. The stimuli included commercially avialable toys incorporating noises (e.g. Fisher Price jack-in-a-box), everyday environmental sounds (e.g. hair dryer) and prerecorded sounds representing the range of frequencies. Audiologists, however, have taken issue with the frequency specificity described in this study (Tucker 1985).

Kershman and Napier stress the importance of the conditions under which observations are made. Hence the children were observed in their own homes, when neither tired nor hungry, as Cairns and Butterfield (1975) have pointed out that the time since an infant's last feed can be a critical variable influencing their auditory functioning. Children with physical impairments were positioned to facilitate their functioning. All children were observed before each stimulus was presented as well as afterwards as illustrated in Figure 1.8, since it was the *change* in their behaviours that was regarded as the critical information.

The strength in Kershman and Napier's study was that it demonstrated that teachers, parents and others could collect reliable observational information enabling any pattern in the individual's auditory responses to emerge. This information could be relayed to the audiologist in any subsequent assessment but could also assist in the planning of individual teaching programmes which might then begin without further delay.

Similar, but less comprehensive, observational procedures used with people with multiple impairments in order to assess their auditory functioning are described by Sebba (1978) and Jones (1984). It is suggested that observational information be used in addition to, rather than instead of, a comprehensive specialist auditory assessment.

A further development in co-operation between specialists and nonspecialists on the assessment of hearing is described by Goetz, Gee and Sailor (1983) and Goetz, Utley, Gee, Baldwin and Sailor (1982)

Figure 1.8: Example of a Completed Auditory Response to Environmental Sounds Sheet

Child's name	John	
Date	21/4	24/4
Describe sound	portable hair dryer	mother's voice calling 'John'
Location of sound (eg. 3 ft. from child or next room)	one foot from John (no air touched him)	five feet to the right of John
What was the child doing when sound occurred?	lying relaxed in reclining seat	being fed, head held by father
Describe response to sound	head turning, eye turning toward sound, face expressed surprise, eye widening	head turned to right, eyes turned to right, smiled, vocalized
Observer	mother	mother and father

Source: Kershman & Napier (1982). 'Systematic Procedures for Eliciting and Recording Responses to Sound Stimuli in Deaf-Blind Multihandicapped Children'. *The Volta Review, 84* (4), 226–37. Reproduced by permission of the Alexander Graham Bell Assn. for the Deaf, Washington, D.C.

who demonstrated that clients with multiple impairments could be taught to produce reliable responses to an auditory stimulus. The training was carried out by classroom staff and involved the pairing of the auditory stimulus with a visual one which was systematically faded once reliable responding had become established. In addition to enabling the audiologists to then carry out more formal testing, this training also provided a method for teaching functional hearing to people who had previously shown no auditory responses. The Goetz *et al.* (1983) study involved students who although having mulitiple impairments were severely rather than profoundly retarded, but there is no reason to suppose that the procedure could not be effectively used with this latter population.

The Assessment of Communication and Prespeech Skills

We have already seen in Volume 1, Chapter 3 how a variety of early aspects of communication can be assessed within tests of sensorimotor development, for example, the vocal imitation scale of the Uzgiris and Hunt (1975) assessment. Suggestions, too, regarding assessment of pragmatic aspects of early communication were further considered in that same chapter. We also find that, as would be expected, communication skills are invariably dealt with in all the global criterion-referenced assessments reviewed earlier in this chapter. Among these assessments, most that concentrate specifically on communication skills are above the level of the population with which we are concerned here. Some assessments have a few items on very early communication skills but are in the main irrelevant to the assessment of children and adults with profound and multiple impairments. Williams (1980) describes approaches to assessing language skills in people with profound retardation but most of his work is concerned with teaching programmes.

The Pre-Verbal Communication Schedule (PVC; Kiernan and Reid 1986) provides a procedure for the assessment of functional communication at the preverbal level, which in practice, makes it applicable to most of the population with profound retardation. It provides a summary of abilities involved in communication and a basis for planning teaching programmes directed at the development of communication skills. It includes a Programme Planning Sheet to assist the staff in this. The schedule is divided into 27 sections covering prerequisites to different forms of communication (e.g. listening, control of hands, etc.), nonverbal communication (e.g. gestures, sound production, etc.), imitation (motor and vocal) and understanding (of nonvocal and vocal and verbal communication). An example of one section, 'Communication Through Pointing', in the nonverbal communication area is given in Figure 1.9. Elsewhere, (Cirrin and Rowland 1985) the importance of detailed assessment of functional communication through nonverbal means has been emphasised. The scoring involves the member of staff or parent stating that the behaviour is observed to occur Usually, Rarely or Never. The percentages on the right hand side refer to the proportions of clients in the standardisation sample who showed this behaviour.

There are two summary scoring sheets included with the schedule, one utilising the lattice method described in relation to the Behaviour Assessment Battery (Kiernan and Jones 1982) earlier in this chapter, and the other summarising specifically some of the items relating to the functional use of communication. The PVC offers a comprehensive, detailed assessment of communication at the earliest level, focusing on items that should be observed during daily activities rather than requiring formal testing. Completion of the entire schedule would certainly be time-consuming but the use of summary scoring methods or of individual

Figure 1.9: A Section from the Pre-Verbal Communication Schedule

---

11. *Communication Through Pointing*
   In this section, one set of items (1, 2, 3, 6) deals with objects which the student *wants to have*, the remaining items (4, 5) deal with objects which the student wishes only to *draw attention* to.

		U R N %
1.	Touches an object he *wants* but does not look at the other person	– – – 81
2.	Touches an object he *wants* and then glances at the other person and object alternatively, until the other person responds. The equivalent of saying *'give me'* or of asking permission	– – – 62
3.	Reaches for objects he *wants* and which are out of reach but without real effort, meanwhile glancing at the object and another person. Again the equivalent of saying *'give me'*.	– – – 58
4.	The student touches objects in order to *draw attention* to them without actually wanting you to do anything except to pay attention. For example he may touch the object and look back and forth between the object and another person until the other person shows that he has paid attention	– – – 42
5.	Points with hand and/or arm to distant objects to *draw attention* to them	– – – 42
6.	Student points with hand and/or arm to distant objects he *wants* whilst looking alternatively at the other person and the object	– – – 40

Comments:

Source: Kiernan and Reid (1986, p. 17).

sections should help overcome this problem. The importance of the area of communication makes this assessment an invaluable contribution.

It has been argued (Warner 1981) that feeding and drinking skills involve the same prerequisite behaviours as early speech. For example, the ability to close the lips and move the tongue are both necessary in order to chew and swallow food but are also vital to making certain speech sounds. It is therefore important to establish appropriate feeding and drinking skills in order to facilitate early speech. Difficulties in the development of these skills tend to be related to such factors as muscle tone, abnormal persistence of reflexes and general physical development. The assessment of feeding and drinking skills has therefore traditionally been carried out by physiotherapists, but this is increasingly becoming an area in which speech therapists are involved.

Warner (1981) constructed a checklist to assess the feeding difficulties

Figure 1.10: Part of a Section from the Early Feeding Checklist

Section IV

CONTROL OF TONGUE AND LIPS FOR FEEDING AND DRINKING

A. FEEDING

> *Even if he is unable to feed himself does your child eat normal family food?*
>
> *that is . . . can he eat solids, either biting an appropriate sized mouthful or taking the food off the spoon or fork with his lips? Can he chew the food* **with lips closed,** *moving his jaw* **round** *as well as up and down? Can he swallow without food escaping from his mouth and without choking?*

YES....... NO........

If your answer is NO check the following . . .

> *Does your child have difficulty sucking or taking food from a spoon because his lips are* **loose and immobile** *and do not close round the teat or spoon?*
>
> OR
>
> *Because the lips curl back in a grimace?*

YES....... NO........

YES....... NO........

> *Does your child have difficulty* **chewing** *because his tongue thrusts forward out of his mouth carrying the food with it?*
>
> OR
>
> *Because the tongue is small and bunched and does not move?*
>
> OR
>
> *Because the tongue is curled back or pushed up against the roof of the mouth?*
>
> OR
>
> *Because the tongue is constantly moving either inside or outside the mouth?*

YES....... NO........

YES....... NO........

YES....... NO........

YES....... NO........

A. FEEDING (cont.)

Does your child only 'chew' in a sucking pattern? *that is . . . mashing the food against the roof of* *the mouth with movements of the jaw up and* *down with very little movement of the tongue?*	YES....... NO........

Does your child chew with tongue movements *but cannot swallow because the lips remain* *open?*	YES....... NO........

Does your child have difficulty with feeding *because he 'bites' the spoon, teat or cup rim* *very hard and cannot release it?*	YES....... NO........

Does your child go into reflex sucking patterns *whenever anything is introduced in his mouth?*	YES....... NO........

Does your child choke very frequently?   YES....... NO........

   . . . on solids **and** fluids   YES....... NO........
   . . . on solids only   YES....... NO........
   . . . on fluids only   YES....... NO........

Does your child seem unaware that food has *been placed in his mouth?*	YES....... NO........

*Can your child **spit** out food he does not like?*	YES....... NO........

Source: Warner (1981 pp. 10 and 11).

and associated problems of oral behaviour encountered in the young child with multiple impairments. The checklist covers general posture and feeding position, movements of the tongue, lips, jaw and soft palate, various problems associated with oral behaviour such as oversensitivity, hygiene and length of feeding time, diet and feeding intervals. An example from the checklist is given in Figure 1.10. This checklist has been widely used by parents and professionals — speech therapists and others. It is linked to a clearly written manual suggesting activities in each area with excellent illustrative diagrams. This will be further discussed in Chapter 6 of this volume.

The Assessment of Vision

In this section we will outline some of the main reasons for assessing vision in people with multiple impairments. We will then review the more widely available procedures used by specialists and those used by nonspecialists. Examples of some of the procedures developed for use by nonspecialists are given in detail.

The high incidence of visual and auditory impairments among people with retardation was noted in Volume 1, Chapter 1. Lawson, Molloy and Miller (1977) found that 70 per cent of their sample of children who were retarded had visual defects compared to 25 per cent in the general school population. Wolf and Anderson (1973) provided further evidence of visual limitations in 50 per cent of children with cerebral palsy. Assessment of visual functioning in people with multiple impairments is therefore likely to reveal some difficulties in many cases.

It is clear that information is required on people's visual acuity in order to design educational programmes that are relevant to their visual and developmental needs. As discussed in Volume 1, Chapter 4, the presence of visual impairments restrict a variety of aspects of development including motor development (Adelson and Fraiberg 1977) which may already be impaired in children with multiple problems. The majority of people with significant visual deficiencies retain some functional vision (Langley and DuBose 1976), but if multiple impairments are present, their limited experiential and cognitive abilites may lead to a tendency for their residual vision to remain largely unused.

Sheridan (1976) has suggested that a distinction can be made between the processes of 'seeing' and 'looking'. 'Seeing' can be considered primarily a physiological process dependent on intact visual mechanisms, whereas 'looking' can be considered primarily a psychological process involving attention to visual stimuli and meaningful interpretation of them.

This suggests the need for assessments of both the structure of the visual organs and the extent to which the person uses their vision.

The justification for assessing visual functioning can hardly be over-stated when vision appears to be the dominant sense (Bower 1974) and it has been suggested that more than 80 per cent of all learning occurs via the visual pathway (Marshall 1977). Visual deficiencies once detected can often be treated and further restrictions on development can thus be avoided.

Assessments Used by Ophthalmologists

The ophthalmologist may carry out a full external and internal examination of the eyes, occasionally using an anaesthetic if required. Examination of the pressure within the eyeball and an examination of its contents by means of an ophthalmoscope may be undertaken, especially if there are indications of defective sight. Full refraction tests may be conducted by an orthoptist. It is beyond the scope of this book to describe these procedures in full but the reader is referred to Bankes (1975) or Markovits (1975).

Information about any structural deficiencies in the eye itself can lead to appropriate treatment to correct them, training to increase the use of residual vision and educational programmes using appropriate materials. If no deficiencies are found but the individual is showing no visual responses, then as with the auditory assessments, it might be assumed to be due to the general attentional and cognitive deficits. However, if the results of an ophthalmology examination indicate no impairments, we still cannot assert with any certainty that the stimulus is reaching the cortex. The only procedures which would establish this in children with profound retardation are the visual evoked response procedures.

Visual Evoked Response Procedures. These procedures are similar to the electrical response audiometry procedures described in the section on hearing, using visual stimuli in a darkened environment rather than auditory stimuli. They are objective tests of neural functioning which measure electrical activity in the visual cortex in response to a light stimulus presented to the eye. Electroretinography, one of the objective electrophysiological tests, measures a mass response of the neural cells of the retina. These procedures have the same disadvantage as the electrical response audiometry ones in that they are expensive, complex, require highly trained expertise to interpret the results and are still not totally reliable.

Sebba (1978) found that children seen by an ophthalmologist sometimes had diagnoses made but no treatment offered due to the extent of other impairments and retardation, which it was argued, made treatment not worthwhile. In some cases, surgery had been performed but very little follow-up appeared to have occurred. It is therefore regarded as crucial to seek the co-operation of an ophthalmologist who is receptive to the idea that treatment of people with multiple impairments would benefit them, even in the face of limited resources.

Other Formal Assessment Procedures

Snellen Chart. The Snellen Chart is the familiar chart used to assess visual acuity in the general population. The person is asked to recognise printed letters or symbols of decreasing size. Defects in visual acuity are then expressed in terms of what the individual sees from a specified distance and at what distance from the chart a normally sighted person would see the same sized letters. The limitations of using this procedure with people with profound retardation obviously relates to whether or not they are able to recognise and communicate recognition of the letters or symbols. In practice, it is of limited use with this population.

Catford Acuity Apparatus. The Catford Drum (Catford and Oliver 1973) projects a series of spots of light which decrease in size until the individual fails to fixate on them. This procedure provides a routine test for evaluating visual acuity and many other procedures exist which similarly measure optokinetic responses in infants and have been used with people with severe handicaps. However, limitations of applying this procedure to people with multiple impairments include difficulties in maintaining the person's fixation of the stimulus, and distinguishing between failure due to poor vision and that due to lack of attention. Furthermore, the dependence of the procedure on a motor response may lead to problems of whether a failure to respond is due to oculomotor defects or visual acuity defects.

Forced Choice Preferential Looking. This technique pioneered by Teller, Morse, Borton and Regal (1974) involves presenting the child with a patterned screen on one side and a blank screen of matched luminance on the other. The side on which the pattern is presented is randomly changed and if the child consistently looks at the pattern this is taken as evidence of visual acuity. It is called 'forced choice' because the observer who records to which side the child looked cannot themselves see on which side the pattern was presented. This procedure can be used with infants of 1–6 months (Atkinson and Braddick 1982) and is therefore useful with older children with very profound retardation.

This technique is similar to the Catford Drum and other optokinetic response procedures but may be considered more objective in its use of independent observers. However, this in itself requires two to three adults, making it a high resource technique. It is also time-consuming and as Nelson, Rubin, Wagner and Breton (1984) point out, it requires an alert and attentive child (rarely a description given for the population of concern here) because of its dependence on a behavioural response.

Stycar Vision Tests. The Stycar Vision Tests developed by Sheridan (1976) have been used extensively to assess visual functioning in children with multiple impairments. The tests were developed specifically for use with children who are developmentally delayed to assess near and distant vision. Langley and DuBose (1976) argue that the Miniature Toys and Rolling Balls Tests are the most useful sub-tests for evaluating vision in children with multiple impairments. The Miniature Toys Test involves naming toys such as a car, plane, doll, chair, etc. instead of the letters or pictures usually used. The Rolling Balls Test consists of a series of graded balls projected at a distance of 10 feet which the child may retrieve after they have been rolled horizontally across the line of vision.

A limitation of using these procedures with children with profound retardation is that they may require too advanced skills for this population. Sheridan suggests that the Miniature Toys Test can be used with children from 21 months and the Rolling Balls Test from 6 months. We have noted in previous chapters that many of the individuals with whom we are concerned are functioning at below the 6-months level. Furthermore, Atkinson and Braddick (1982) argue that the balls are not the appropriate stimulus for testing visual acuity and a further possible problem concerns the noise made by the balls rolling. Both tests involve motor skills that the child with multiple impairments may be unable to perform.

New York Flashcard Vision Test. This test developed by Faye (1968) to assess visual acuity in people with multiple impairments, involves presenting the individual with flashcards of three symbols — a heart, a house and an umbrella of varying sizes. The person is required to give any consistent verbal or manual label to the symbols or to point to large matching symbols. Aside from the obvious question as to why these particular objects were chosen, this test is considered suitable for children from 27 months which is clearly developmentally more advanced than many of the individuals with whom we are concerned.

Assessments Used by Nonspecialists

Some of the procedures described above have been used or adapted for use by nonspecialists such as teachers, nurses and parents. However, they can still be considered to represent formal assessment procedures. Langley and DuBose (1976) have stressed the need for informal but systematic assessment procedures which can be used by nonspecialists in a similar way to that discussed above in relation to hearing. Hence, important, practical information about a person's visual functioning on a daily basis can both inform the development of individual programmes and assist the specialist in making their assessments. Bell (1983) describes various assessments for use by the nonspecialist including her own observation list and the functional vision screening procedure developed by Langley and DuBose (1976) and Langley (1980). This latter procedure has been further adapted by Sebba (1978) for use with people with profound retardation and multiple impairments.

Bell's Observation List is not a published assessment with a manual, scoring sheets or test materials but a description of the information that should be recorded during observations by a 'significant person' on how the person is using her or his vision. Bell (1983) states that specialist assessments, although necessary to provide information on a child's eye defects, visual acuity and visual field, are unlikely to provide information on the ways in which the child uses vision or about the motivation to do so. Periods of systematic observation during the normal daily routine may pick up on the subtle behaviour changes which may indicate a visual response in a person who is profoundly handicapped. Bell's guidelines for observation are given in Figure 1.11.

From these observations Bell suggests drawing up a 'summary and action sheet' which must include the specification of the conditions under which optimum use of vision occurs and the teaching objective in the area of visual skills. There are no reliability figures reported in Bell's article but this procedure could easily be subjected to a similar attempt to establish reliability between various staff and parents as was reported above in relation to Kershman and Napier's hearing checklist.

The Visual Assessment Checklist from Sebba (1978) illustrated in Figure 1.12 is based on an assessment of functional vision devised by Langley and DuBose (1976) and Langley (1980) who attempted to produce an informal assessment that could be used by teachers with children who are severely retarded. The assessment is considered 'informal' in contrast to the more 'formal' approach adopted by ophthal-

Figure 1.11: Bell's Guidelines for Observing Visual Behaviour

1. The extent to which he is 'visually curious'. Does he look at desired or new items or does he touch, taste or smell them in preference?
2. The extent of his visual interest in people. Does he look at people's faces? Does he watch people as they move around the room? Is there anyone in particular he likes looking at?
3. The kind of objects he will look at. Is interest affected by their purpose, size, colour, shape, pattern or by their appeal to his other senses.
4. The distance at which visual attention is given most readily.
5. The preferred angle of view.
6. The preferred or dominant eye or side.
7. The extent to which vision is used to direct and monitor reach and grasp. The accuracy of the reach in terms of both distance and direction.
8. The speed with which he notices things to the sides when he is looking straight ahead.
9. If mobile, the extent to which he avoids or bumps into obstacles. Is this related to their size, position, colour or their familiarity?
10. The effect of place or time on his willingness to use sight. Is it related to motivation, lighting, comfort or to the competition from other stimuli? Does he use vision to the same extent at home and at school?
11. The negative signs. The things which he consistently fails to see. The presence of mannerisms e.g. eye-poking, head-weaving or light gazing which may indicate loss of sight.

Source: Bell (1983 p. 17).

mologists or standardised testing procedures, but it utilises systematic evaluation. Sebba selected some of the earlier items from the list devised by Langley and DuBose and thus scaled down the assessment to suit children with more profound retardation. It is designed to assist staff in systematically observing basic visual responses in people with severe and profound retardation for whom more formal testing procedures may not be suitable. It is not intended to be used in the place of examination by an eye specialist but to assist staff working daily with the client to plan individual programmes.

The checklist requires no complex materials or procedures and can be carried out in a corner of a classroom if necessary although a darkened room is likely to maximise responses. Objects must include a light source and should be selected for clarity, flourescent colours being particularly useful. Furthermore, in all but the last item of the checklist which is on visual response to sounds, the objects should not be sound-producing since this might confuse the responses.

The assessment consists of nine items but all the items need not be completed in one session. They are concerned with the presence or absence of the basic visual responses. The pupils are observed and any

Figure 1.12: A Section from Sebba's 1978 Adaptation of Langley and DuBose (1976), for People with Profound and Multiple Impairments

---

1. *Pupil Reaction*
   a) Do the pupils constrict and dilate continually when the person is in constant light?
   If they do, this suggests a visual defect and you should move to question 2.
   If they do not:-

	Yes	No

   b) Direct torch light into the eyes from approximately 45 cms
   Do pupils constrict to light?
   Do pupils dilate when light is removed?

	R	L

2. *Muscle Balance* (assessing for a squint)
   Hold light 45 cms from mid point between the two eyes.
   Is the light reflected simultaneously in the centre of each pupil?
   If not, a squint may be observed.

	R	L

3. *Blink Reaction*
   From behind the client, move your hand over their eyes from their chin to their forehead approximately 5 cm away from their face. Pause, and repeat 5 times. Tick each time they blink.

1	2	3	4	5	6

4. *Visual Field*
   Flash the light on and off from approximately 45 cms, above, below and to the left and right of the client. Tick if attention is given to the light eg. eyes fix on light, client reaches for light. Repeat.

	Above	Below	Left	Right
1				
2				

5. *Peripheral Vision*
   Bring the light from behind the client, slowly into the left and then the right visual field. Tick if the client turns their head or eyes to the light when the torch is in line with the lateral position of the eye. Repeat 3 times.

	Head or eye turn to right	Head or eye turn to left
1		
2		
3		
4		

6. *Visual Field Preference*
   Present two identical non-sound producing toys simultaneously in the right and left visual fields. Tick the side to which the client looks first. Repeat 5 times.

	1	2	3	4	5	6
Left						
Right						
None						

---

continual constricting and dilating of the pupil (known as hippus) is noted as this may indicate a visual impairment. The penlight torch is then shone into the eyes and constriction of the pupils is noted, followed by dilation of the pupils when the light is removed. This response to light is a basic involuntary response. The light is then held directly in the midline and observation of its reflection simultaneously in the centre of each pupil is noted. If it is not in the centre of each pupil a muscle imbalance or squint is suggested. An attempt is then made to elicit the blink reaction by passing the hand over the person's face from behind the person's head. The blink reflex indicates some light perception, and possibly some object perception, although Bower (1974) has noted that both visual and air displacement aspects are involved in eliciting blink responses by objects moving in front of the face. The air displacement caused by passing the hand horizontally over the person's face is far less than that caused by a directly approaching object from the front. The procedure is repeated five times to see if any consistency emerges, but the blink reflex is regarded as present if observed only twice.

The visual field of the person is tested by repeatedly flashing the penlight torch on and off above, below and to the left and right of the child. Any attention to the light or apparent fixation in the various different positions is recorded, and the procedure is done with the individual in both lying and sitting positions. Peripheral vision is assessed by bringing the light slowly round in a horizontal plane from behind the person's head until it is in line with the lateral portion of the eye at which point any visual attention to the light is noted. These two items testing the range of the visual field and peripheral vision may reveal discrepancies between areas to which the person attends. This may indicate specific impairments which could therefore provide a basis for referral to an ophthalmologist, but also provides important information about the position in which visual stimuli are presented to the individual.

Visual field preference is tested by presenting two identical nonsound-producing toys simultaneously in the left and right visual field and noting which toy is attended to first. This is repeated five times to estimate consistency of responses. The information derived from this item may support or contradict that derived from the item on the range of the visual field.

Eye preference is noted by the same cover test as that used by some ophthalmologists. Each eye is covered in turn, without actual contact, while the person is attending to an object, and any resistence is noted. This is repeated three times with each eye to estimate consistency in responses elicited. The eye preference test can indicate limited or no vision in one eye, since the person is unlikely to resist having that eye covered but may strongly resist the covering of the functional eye.

The next item involves detailed observation of the individual's ability to follow a moving stimulus with his or her eyes. A strong stimulus (light) is moved in the horizontal, vertical and circular directions. This is one of the earliest visual responses and provides a useful basis for task selection when attempting to increase the use of residual vision.

The final item is the only item in which sound is incorporated. Two identical sound-producing toys are held approximately 12 inches apart in the individual's visual field equidistant from midline. Each toy is shaken in turn and an eye movement indicating shifts in attention to the appropriate toy is noted. This is repeated three times to estimate consistency of the response observed. This visual response of shifting attention from one item to another represents a more advanced use of vision.

It should be noted that the visual field and tracking items require administration in both sitting and lying positions. The reasons for this are that the responses in these two positions are sometimes reported as being different. Thus, Hisley (1978) has noted that the lying position can interfere with vision due to the pressure exerted on the back of the head. Fieber (1977) has noted differences in visual perception in various different positions in children with multiple impairments. Furthermore Bower (1974) has suggested that visual assessments should always be carried out in a sitting position since the infant may not be fully awake in a lying position. It is therefore considered worthwhile to compare the responses obtained in these two positions. No formal evaluation or inter-rater reliabilities have been carried out on this checklist but informal feedback from teachers would suggest it was a useful basic tool for informal but systematic assessment of visual functioning.

Conclusion

This chapter has covered some of the components of an interdisciplinary assessment for the individual with profound and multiple impairments. In particular, we have stressed the need for specialist assessments in conjunction with transfer of some skills from specialists to direct contact personnel to enable continuous criterion-referenced assessment to take place. Finally, we have suggested procedures in each area that can be carried out by nonspecialists in order to assist the specialists and to inform day-to-day intervention. In the next chapter we turn to what the intervention might involve.

References

Adelson, E. and Fraiberg, S. (1977) 'Gross Motor Development' in S. Fraiberg (ed.), *Insights from the Blind,* Souvenir Press, London

Atkinson, J. and Braddick, O. (1982) 'Assessment of Visual Acuity in Infancy and Early Childhood', *Acta Ophthalmologica Supplement, 157,* 18–26

Bankes, J.L.K. (1975) 'The Ophthalmologists Role in Multidisciplinary Assessment of Developmentally Handicapped Children', *Child: Care, Health and Development, 1,* 325–33

Barratt, H. (1980) 'Electric Response Audiometry and its Application to the Assessment of Hearing in Children', *Journal of the British Association of Teachers of the Deaf, 4,* 4

Bell, J. (1983) 'Assessment of Visual Ability in the Profoundly Handicapped', *National Association of Deaf Blind Rubella Handicapped Newsletter, 29,* 16–17

Bobath, K. and Bobath, B. (1956) 'The Diagnosis of Cerebral Palsy in Infancy', *Archives of Disease in Childhood, 31,* 408–14

Bower, T. (1974) *Development in Infancy,* Freeman, London

Cairns, G.F. and Butterfield, E.C. (1975) 'Assessing Infants' Auditory Functioning' in B.Z. Friedlander, G.M. Steritt and F.G.E. Kirk (eds.), *Exceptional Infant: Vol. 3,* Brunner/Mazel Inc., New York

Catford, G.V. and Oliver, A. (1973) 'Development of Visual Acuity', *Archives of Disease in Childhood, 48,* 47–50

Cirrin, F.M. and Rowland, C.M. (1985) 'Communicative Assessment of Nonverbal Youths with Severe/Profound Mental Retardation', *Mental Retardation, 23,* 52–62

Collins, M.T. and Rudolph, J.M. (1975) 'A Manual for the Assessment of a Deaf-Blind Multiply-Handicapped Child', unpublished manuscript, Michigan

Cunningham, C. and McArthur, K. (1981) 'Hearing Loss and Treatment in Young Down's Syndrome Children', *Child: Care, Health and Development, 7,* 357–74

DuBose, R.F. (1977) 'Evaluation and Instruction of Severely and Profoundly Handicapped' in J. Cronin (ed.), *The Severely and Profoundly Handicapped Child,* State Board of Education, Illinois

DuBose, R.F. and Langley, M.B. (1977) *The Developmental Activities Screening Inventory,* Teaching Resources, Boston

Faye, E.E. (1968) 'A New Visual Acuity Test for Partially-Sighted Non-Readers', *Journal of Paediatric Ophthalmology, 5,* 210–12

Felce, D., Jenkins, J., de Kock, U. and Mansell, J. (1986) *The Bereweeke Skill-Teaching System: Goal Setting Checklist for Adults,* NFER-Nelson, Windsor

Fieber, N. (1977) 'Sensorimotor Cognitive Assessment and Curriculum for the Multihandicapped Child' in J. Cronin (ed.), *The Severely and Profoundly Handicapped Child,* State Board of Education, Illinois

Freedman, D.G. (1964) 'Smiling in Blind Infants and the Issue of Innate Versus Acquired', *Journal of Child Psychology and Psychiatry and Allied Disciplines, 5,* 171–84

Goetz, L., Gee, K. and Sailor, W. (1983) 'Crossmodal Transfer of Stimulus Control: Preparing Students with Severe Multiple Disabilities for Audiological Assessment', *Journal of the Association for Persons with Severe Handicap, 8,* 3–13

Goetz, L., Utley, B., Gee, K., Baldwin, M. and Sailor, W. (1982) *Auditory Assessment and Programming Manual for Severely Handicapped and Deaf-Blind Students,* The Association for the Severely Retarded, Seattle

Gunstone, C. (1979, revised 1985) *Checklists used at Anson House Preschool Project*, Barnardo's, Barkingside

Gunzburg, H.C. (1963) *Progress Assessment Charts*, NAMH, London

Hisley, T. (1978) 'Classification and Assessment of the Special Care Child', unpublished paper presented at the Royal Manchester Children's Hospital to a meeting on 'Education of the Special Care Child', 31 January 1978

Hogg, J. (1978) 'The Development of a Fine Motor Skill Assessment Battery for Use with Mentally Handicapped Preschool Children', unpublished report, Hester Adrian Research Centre, University of Manchester, Manchester

Holt, K.S. (1965) *Assessment of Cerebral Palsy*, Lloyd-Luke, London

Holt, K.S. (1975) (ed.), *Movement and Child Development*, Heinemann, London

Jeffree, D.M. and McConkey, R. (1976) *P.I.P. Development Charts*, Hodder and Stoughton, Sevenoaks

Jones, L. (1984) 'Curriculum Evaluation for the Profoundly Retarded Multiply Handicapped Child', unpublished manuscript, Lea Castle Hospital, Kidderminster

Kershman, S.M. and Napier, D. (1982) 'Systematic Procedures for Eliciting and Recording Responses to Sound Stimuli in Deaf-Blind Multihandicapped Children', *The Volta Review, 84*, 226–37

Kiernan, C.C. and Jones, M. (1982) *The Behaviour Assessment Battery*, NFER-Nelson, Windsor

Kiernan, C.C. and Reid, B. (1986) *The Pre-Verbal Communication Schedule*, NFER-Nelson, Windsor

Langley, M.B. and DuBose, R.F. (1976) 'Functional Vision Screening for Severely Handicapped Children', *The New Outlook*, October 1976, 346–50
—— (1980) *Functional Vision Inventory*, Stoelting Co., Chicago

Lawson, L.J., Molloy, J.S. and Miller, M. (1977) 'A Technique for Appraising the Vision of Mentally Retarded Children', in P. Mittler (ed.), *Research to Practice in Mental Retardation: Vol. 11: Education and Training*, University Park Press, Baltimore

Levitt, S. (1982) *Treatment of Cerebral Palsy and Motor Delay*, Blackwell, Oxford

Mansell, J., Felce, D., Jenkins, J., and Flight, C. (1984) *Bereweeke Skill Teaching System*, NFER-Nelson, Windsor

Markovits, A.S. (1975) 'Ophthalmic Screening of the Mentally Defective', *Annals of Ophthalmology, 7*, 846–48

Marshall, G.H. (1977) *The Eyes and Vision*, Exhall Grange School, Warwickshire

Molnar, G.E. and Alexander, J. (1983) 'Strength Development in Retarded Children: A Comparative Study on the Effect of Intervention', in J. Hogg and P.J. Mittler (eds.), *Advances in Mental Handicap Research: Vol. 2*, Wiley, London

Nelson, L.B., Rubin, S.E., Wagner, R.S. and Breton, M.E. (1984) 'Developmental Aspects in the Assessment of Visual Function in Young Children', *Pediatrics 73*, 375–81

Nihira, K., Foster, R., Shellhaas, M., and Leland, H. (1974) *AAMD Adaptive Behavior Scale*, American Association on Mental Deficiency, Washington, DC.

Perkins, E.A., Taylor, P.D. and Capie, A.C.M. (1976) *Developmental Checklists*, British Institute of Mental Handicap, Kidderminster

Popovich, D. (1977) *A Prescriptive Behavioral Checklist for the Severely and Profoundly Handicapped: Vol. 1*, University Park Press, Baltimore

Popovich, D. (1981) *A Prescriptive Behavioral Checklist for the Severely and Profoundly Handicapped: Vols. 2 and 3*, University Park Press, Baltimore

Popovich, D. and Laham, S.L. (1981) *The Adaptive Behavior Curriculum: Vol. 1*, Brookes Publishing Co., Baltimore

Presland, J. (1982) *Paths to Mobility in 'Special Care'*, British Institute of Mental Handicap, Kidderminster

Sebba, J. (1978) 'A System for Assessment and Intervention for Preschool Profoundly Retarded Multiply Handicapped Children', unpublished M.Ed. thesis, University of Manchester, Manchester

Shearer, D.E., Billingsley, J., Frohman, A., Hilliard, J., Johnson, F., and Shearer, M.S. (1972) *The Portage Guide to Early Education*, CESA, Wisconsin

Sheridan, M.D. (1976) *Manual for the Sycar Vision Tests*, NFER, Windsor

Simon, G.B. (1981) *The Next Step on the Ladder*, British Institute of Mental Handicap, Kidderminster

Taylor, I.G. (1968) 'The Partially Hearing Spastic Child' in. J. Loring (ed.), *Assessment of the Cerebral Palsied Child for Education*, Spastics Society, London

Teller, D.Y., Morse, R., Borton, R. and Regal, D. (1974) 'Visual Acuity for Vertical and Diagonal Gratings in Human Infants', *Vision Research, 14*, 1433–9

Tucker, I. (1985) personal communication

Tucker, I. and Nolan, M. (1984) *Educational Audiology*, Croom Helm, London, Sydney, Dover, N.H.

Uzgiris, I.C. and Hunt, J. McV (1975) *Assessment in Infancy: Ordinal Scales of Psychological Development*, University of Illinois Press, Urbana

Warner, J. (1981) *Helping the Handicapped Child with Early Feeding*, Winslow Press, Buckingham

Webb, R.C., Schultz, B. and McMahill, J. (1977) 'The Glenwood Awareness Manipulation and Posture Scale', unpublished manuscript, Glenwood State Hospital School, Iowa

Williams, C. (1980) *Towards Teaching Communication Skills*, British Institute of Mental Handicap, Kidderminster

Williams, C. (1982a) *The Star Profile: Social Training Achievement Record*, British Institute of Mental Handicap, Kidderminster

Williams, C. (1982b) 'Deaf not Daft: The Deaf in Subnormality Hospitals', *Special Education: Forward Trends, 9*, 26–8

Wolf, J.M. and Anderson, R.M. (1973) *The Multiply Handicapped Child*, Charles C. Thomas, Springfield

Woods, P. and Parry, R. (1981) 'Pethna: Tailor-Made Toys for the Severely Retarded and Multiply Handicapped', *Apex, 9*, 53–6

2 TEACHING AND THERAPEUTIC METHODS

Introduction

In this chapter the current methods used to teach people with profound and multiple impairments will be reviewed. Initially consideration will be given to what constitutes a curriculum for this population and what might be the objectives of such a curriculum. The elements of the curriculum will be discussed including curriculum content, teaching methods, resources and environmental considerations. The sources from which a curriculum for people with profound and multiple handicaps can be derived will be outlined with specific examples of materials currently available. Finally holistic approaches such as those implied by conductive education and the Doman methods will be reviewed.

What is a Curriculum for People with Profound and Multiple Handicaps?

In recent years in special education there seems to have been far more interest in teaching methods than in the content of what to teach. Historically, the essentials were selected from the elementary school curriculum, the demands in each subject were lowered and teaching was arranged to involve shorter periods of concentration (Wilson 1981). The emphasis has shifted from factual knowledge to social competence and more specifically to future needs such as everyday living skills. Hence, whereas in ordinary education the 'curriculum' is a term which may be defined as 'all the opportunities for learning provided by a school', it is arguable that for pupils with severe and profound learning difficulties the definition should be expanded to include all opportunities for learning 'in' or 'out' of school (Committee on Special Educational Needs (COSPEN) 1984). More specifically the curriculum consists of a framework of goals within which skills, teaching methods and recording are specified.

The 1970 Education Act in England and Wales and similar legislation in Scotland transferred responsibility for the education of children with severe and profound learning difficulties from the health authorities to the education authorities. Since then, compulsory education for all children however profound and multiple their difficulties has been a legal requirement. Similarly, since Public Law 94–142 was introduced in the USA in 1975, educational programming for all children has been mandatory. Hence, there is official recognition of the philosophical position that every child has a right to an education. However, McLean (1984) found that those whose handicaps were most severe were still not receiving education in hospitals in Scotland and what was received was less well resourced in terms of classrooms and qualified teachers than was available to those with less severe handicaps. Furthermore, the controversy over whether people with profound impairments can benefit from programming or should instead receive enriching activities is still raging, especially in the USA. Stainback and Stainback's (1983) review of evidence regarding the educability of people with profound retardation strongly supports the effectiveness of teaching. A number of legal cases in the USA have set precedents supporting mandatory programming for even those with the most profound impairments, as we have discussed in more detail elsewhere (Hogg 1985).

There is a paucity of research findings supporting or challenging the effectiveness of programming with this population. Hotte, Monroe, Philbrood and Scarlata (1984) demonstrated that the lowest functioning people (defined by a Social Maturity Quotient (SMQ) of less than 10) do not benefit from intensive programming, (average 27 hours/week) compared to the slightly less profoundly handicapped (defined by a SMQ of 10–19). One question that arises from this study and mentioned previously in Volume 1, Chapter 7 is whether the gains made by those who are lowest functioning are too small to be apparent on standardised tests. Furthermore, the differences between the lower and higher functioning groups were only just statistically significant. We shall see in subsequent chapters of this book that successful attempts have been made to teach specific skills to even those whose impairments are most profound.

The Objectives of a Curriculum for People with Profound and Multiple Handicaps

The objectives of education for all people would seem to be concerned with developing independence, increased opoortunities and socialisation. The objectives of education for people with profound and multiple handicaps might be considered similarly. It is argued that it is through the curriculum that the educational process can be enacted (Bailey 1983).

The curriculum first and foremost provides the framework for all work done in the school. This could be extended to other settings such as hospital wards, social education centres or group homes in which a framework of all activities is still a necessary requirement for the 'education' of the people concerned. We should not assume that the word 'curriculum' applies only to schools since as we have stated 'education' for people with profound and multiple handicaps may take place anywhere and everywhere.

In providing a framework, the curriculum should be a clear public statement of the aims and objectives of the agency concerned. It should provide guidelines for staff, help to plan teaching of individual skills and to relate individual work being carried out simultaneously in different areas by providing an overall plan for each individual child or adult. In addition the framework provided by a curriculum should ensure relatively clear induction of new staff into the overall plan operating in that agency but also help maintain continuity and progression (Wilson 1981).

A clear curriculum offers accurate information for professionals involved with individuals on a consultancy basis, current information on skills for case conferences and specific information on progress for parents and staff alike. Parents can use the curriculum to assist in the identification of areas in which they can offer assistance, specific expertise and consistency. It is perhaps for some of these reasons that some of the local education authorities in England and Wales insist that their schools all have written curricula. However, this does not necessarily ensure that each teacher actually works from the curriculum as, for example, it may remain shut away in the filing cabinet.

Elements of the Curriculum

This section is divided into curricular content, teaching methods and strategies, aspects of the teaching environment and curricular resources.

Curricular Content

How would we set about devising a curriculum for people with profound and multiple handicaps had we not inherited an academic framework which some would consider inappropriate for this population. 'Formal' education is to a greater extent concerned with the acquisition of factual knowledge and the development of analytical skills. This has provided the basis for the 'core' curriculum which might include language, number, reading, etc. and has been distinguished from the 'peripheral' curriculum which might include creative, aesthetic and practical activities and knowledge about the environment. A similar distinction has been drawn in the special education curriculum by Tansley and Gulliford (1960) and was further developed by Brennan (1974) who referred to 'Education for Mastery' (core) and 'Education for Awareness' (peripheral). In both cases the 'Education for Awareness' or peripheral curriculum was seen as no less important than the 'Education for Mastery' (core) and it was recognised that they were closely linked and interdependent.

Traditionally, in both mainstream and special education, the core curriculum is always covered by the school whereas aspects of the peripheral curriculum, for example some knowledge of the environment, is assumed to be gained outside the school. COSPEN (1984) has argued that for pupils with severe and profound learning difficulties, the formal school programme must include the teaching of skills which pupils in general education are assumed to acquire before or outside school, even though they may be further developed in schools. These skills might include basic communication, and some self-help skills such as feeding, dressing, etc.

It is this requirement of the curriculum for pupils with profound learning difficulties that leads to the argument that the curriculum should be turned inside out, the peripheral becoming the core and vice versa. The core curriculum becomes the basic understanding of the world including communication and daily living skills whereas traditional 'academic' activities like 'reading', writing, etc., become the periphery. This process needs careful monitoring to ensure that pupils with severe and profound difficulties do not spend their school day exclusively increasing their awareness of the environment through shopping trips, drama and so on, at the expense of more 'formal' educational opportunities. Perhaps for this reason the Rectory Paddock School (1983) curriculum has kept the more traditional definition of a 'core' curriculum which includes mathematical skills, communication and literacy and has termed other activites including practical and personal/social conduct as the applied curriculum. In Hegarty, Pocklington and Bradley's (1982) description of the Rectory Paddock School curriculum in action they reported that four mornings a week are spent on the core curriculum and the rest of the time on the applied curriculum, thus operationalising the point made by Brennan and others that the peripheral (applied) curriculum was no less important. In Chapters 3, 4, 5 and 6 we discuss the core curricular areas of cognitive, communication, motor and self-help skills in more detail.

One approach to curriculum planning and development suggested by Wilson (1981) involves identification of the educational needs of the child within three categories: the experiences, e.g. aesthetic, scientific, etc.; the skills, e.g. reading, measurement, etc.; and the attitudes, e.g. self-discipline, sensitivity, etc. These categories of needs are distinguished from the curricular components offered by the school such as English, Science and work experience. The model is used to indicate which activities are contributing to which need. This model would seem to be applicable to even the lowest functioning children since their needs could be similarly classified and an attempt made to match the activities offered by the special school, centre or hospital to them. For example, the needs category of mobility would be matched to the curriculum offering motor skills.

The model outlined by Crawford (1980) and later developed by Gardner, Murphy and Crawford (1983) is shown in Figure 2.1. It is similar to Wilson's approach in that it specifies the first step in curriculum development as identification of the 'core' areas of the curriculum which involves consideration of the needs of the client group and the main areas of teaching required to meet those needs. Applications of this model are fully described in the Walsall Education Department (undated) curriculum and have been successfully used with pupils with severe and profound learning difficulties for whom it was designed.

Figure 2.1: Summary of the Skills Analysis Model

STEP ONE:	Identify CORE areas of the curriculum.
STEP TWO:	Subdivide core areas into their COMPONENT parts.
STEP THREE	Write TARGETS for each component.
STEP FOUR:	ORDER targets.
STEP FIVE:	Write PROGRAMME designed to teach target skills.
STEP SIX:	Devise an on-going ASSESSMENT and RECORD-KEEPING System.

Source: From Gardner, J., Murphy, J. and Crawford, N. (1983), *The Skills Anaylsis Model,* British Institute of Medical Handicap, Kidderminster. Reproduced by kind permission of the publishers BIMH Publications.

COSPEN (1984) identified four core areas of the curriculum for pupils with profound learning difficulties: Language and Concept Formation; Motor Skills; Self-Help Skills; and Relationships. These four, otherwise labelled as cognitive, communication, motor skills and self-help, are perhaps those areas defined as priorities by most staff and parents concerned with people with profound and multiple impairments. They appear in most published curricula aimed at this population (see for example Popovich and Laham 1981, Simon 1981 and Wehman 1979) and thereby provide the areas we discuss more fully in later chapters of this book. A curriculum manual written for staff and parents working with deaf-blind children (California State Department of Education 1976) has a similar emphasis with the communication section concerned mainly with the use of American Sign Language. Most curricula designed for this population have additional core areas such as social skills, although the parameters, the labels and the overlap between areas are somewhat arbitrary. Baker, Jupp, Myland and Thurlow (1981) suggest communication, movement and cognitive skills as the three core areas but all sensory perception skills are subsumed under cognitive skills in their curriculum, which is a common practice.

It is clear that although specifying content areas for a whole school or centre may be useful, within each area individual targets for each child will vary considerably. Later in this chapter, we shall review specific curricula in more detail but as we have seen there are plenty of attempts not to limit the education of people with profound and multiple impairments to 'enrichment activities' alone. Furthermore, we may define a core curriculum for this population which includes not only the more educationally 'formal' cognitive skills (even if at a lower level) but also mobility and communication which necessarily involves programming by therapists and teachers together. The role of therapists has therefore become more educational and their activities can no longer be regarded as part of an alternative 'enrichment' programme.

Teaching Methods and Strategies

The distinction between teaching methods and curriculum content is to some extent arbitrary in that specific content areas may also be seen as methods. For example, the content area painting could be regarded as a method of teaching fine motor skills. This section will review some of the teaching techniques found to be most effective with people with profound handicaps. Many of these techniques are derived from the behavioural theory of learning which, as we shall see in the review of curricula (pp. 72–81), is also the basis for many of the curriculum models used with this population. The use of group and individual instruction will also be discussed.

Common elements of behavioural approaches to teaching people with profound handicaps include the use of precisely defined targets or objectives, task analysis and chaining, shaping, reinforcement, prompts, imitation, errorless learning techniques and recording methods or evaluation. We have argued elsewhere that these techniques, although powerful, still have limitations with those whose impairments are most profound and should be used cautiously and critically. There is little doubt that they are being extensively used, Hegarty *et al.* (1982) having noted the use particularly of specific objectives, task analysis and record-keeping in schools for pupils with severe and profound learning difficulties.

An excellent review of the literature on the use of teaching techniques with children with profound learning difficulties is provided in Presland (1980). Books which give details on the practical application of these techniques include Gardner *et al.* (1983), Kiernan, Jordan and Saunders (1978), Kiernan (1981), McBrien and Foxen (1981), Perkins, Taylor and Capie (1980), Jeffree, McConkey and Hewson (1977) and Ainscow and Tweddle (1981), although these do not relate exclusively to children with profound learning difficulties. Individual techniques are described in detail by some authors, for example Ainscow and Tweddle (1981) on objectives and Haring (1977) on recording.

Objectives or Targets. Ainscow and Tweddle (1981) have argued that the teaching of basic skills to slow learning children should involve developing the curriculum in terms of objectives. These objectives demand that the teacher knows precisely what the pupil will be able to do at the end of teaching that particular activity. The objective has three parts: a statement of the observable behaviour the pupil should demonstrate following instruction; a statement of any important conditions under which the behaviour should occur such as assistance, circumstances of time, place or persons present; and criterion for success, that is, a statement of how many times the individual must perform the task correctly before we are convinced that it has been learnt and are ready to move on to the next task.

This objectives approach is even more relevant with individuals with severe and profound learning difficulties, since arguably the more impaired the individual, the more precisely defined the teaching should be in order to be quite clear on the purpose of the activity. This is, to some extent, the opposing position to that which suggests the provision of a stimulating and enriching environment described in the previous section. The objectives-based curriculum has been more commonly used in schools for pupils with severe learning difficulties in recent years and is beginning to be adopted as an approach in other types of special schools and increasingly as a curriculum model for meeting special needs in ordinary schools. Reasons for the popularity with teachers of this approach are described in detail in Ainscow and Tweddle (1981) but include the assistance it provides in planning and the link to criterion-based assessment which, as discussed in Chapter 1 of this volume, has also become increasingly popular. Furthermore, providing clear objectives for every individual and in some cases involving the person in the choice of objectives appears to foster positive attitudes in the individuals and teachers and perhaps, thereby, to result in greater progress. It enables more precise records and evaluation to take place, providing a basis for information exchange with parents and other professionals.

Task Analysis. Task analysis is perhaps the best-known teaching technique in special education. It involves the breaking down of a target or objective into smaller steps, in which each step is intended to be achievable in a short time. The same objective can be broken down into more smaller steps or fewer larger ones depending on the level of the individual. The steps are sometimes taught in the order in which they are written or sometimes in reverse order. These are termed forward and backward chaining respectively as the steps represent the 'links' in the 'chain'. Backward chaining, in which teaching begins with the last step, is often used to ensure the task is completed and the individual rewarded. For example, if an individual was being taught to eat with a spoon, the steps might include grasps spoon, scoops food, lifts loaded spoon to mouth, puts spoon in mouth, takes food off spoon, chews and swallows food. In this case teaching on the last step first, ensures the individual gets the food which we shall assume is something he or she likes.

Reinforcement. Reinforcements are anything a person will work for, or, in behavioural theory terms, anything that increases the chances of the behaviour being repeated. An excellent description of using them is provided in Kiernan (1981). Chapter 9 of Volume 1 reviewed the work on the use of reinforcements with people with profound learning difficulties (see for examples Murphy and Doughty 1977, and Remington, Foxen and Hogg 1977) and it is clear that there are more difficulties encountered in identifying suitable reinforcements for this population than for less severely impaired people. However, Pace *et al.* (1985) report that reinforcers for which individuals with profound retardation have demonstrated preference will be more effective than nonpreferred ones. Moreover, the use of reinforcements should be carefully considered, in particular, issues such as providing a variety of them, systematic use and timing (see Kiernan *et al.* 1978). Generally, as suggested in Kiernan (1981), the use of consumable and material reinforcements should be paired with social and verbal reinforcements to maximise the possiblity of eventually using only the latter. This is suggested because of the practical and in some cases ethical difficulties of using consumable and material reinforcements especially in group settings. As pointed out elsewhere in the literature, to be effective reinforcements should be consistent and immediate.

Shaping involves reinforcing successively closer approximations to the target behaviour. This technique can be particularly useful in relation to teaching speech since any attempts need to be encouraged and possibilities for the use of physical assistance in teaching these skills is somewhat limited. Examples of this are again given in the practical manuals referenced above.

Prompting. In situations in which the behaviour does not currently occur at all, it may be necessary to give some assistance rather than wait until the behaviour occurs in order to reward it. This assistance or prompt can be physical, gestural or verbal as long as it results in the target behaviour. Prompted responses are rewarded and the prompts are faded out as quickly as possible to ensure the child does not become dependent on them but that the target behaviour is still reached. Murphy and Doughty (1977) provide one of the many examples of using prompts with people with profound and multiple impairments. They demonstrated the use of physical guidance to teach simple arm movements.

More recently, interest has been shown (Halle and Touchette 1986) in using delayed prompting in preference to fading as a method of transferring stimulus control. The prompt is delayed in order to give the individual an opportunity to respond appropriately prior to it being given. Once the response precedes the prompt every time, the prompt is no longer required. The advantage of this procedure over traditional fading procedures is that it shifts the control from the stimuli provided by the instructor to the stimuli inherent in the task or situation. It can be used within the individual's natural environment to promote generalisation by transferring the control from contrived prompts to stimuli which exist within the daily routines. The clearest examples of applications of delayed prompting procedures are in the area of teaching functional language. The conventional procedure of producing food, drink or an activity and getting the individual to provide a verbal label is replaced by delaying the presentation of the item until it has been requested. An application of the delayed prompting procedure with children who are profoundly retarded is described in Chapter 4 of this volume.

Imitation. Imitation is a kind of prompting in that a model of the behaviour is being provided for the child to copy. Most children learn to imitate spontaneously but those who have profound impairments may need to be taught to imitate. Baer, Peterson and Sherman (1967) suggest that imitation is a powerful technique for children with limited skills both in the process of socialisation in general and in the development of communication in particular. These authors provide a full description of imitation training which includes the desirability of initially using motor actions which the individual is already able to do. Choosing actions which only require one of the teacher's hands for the model, enables the model to be maintained as long as necessary and the teacher's other hand to be available for prompting. Initially, the action is exaggerated by the model and fading then involves providing a less accentuated model and decreasing the time the model remains available. Thus, the individual learns to copy from 'memory'. Once previously learned physical actions can be successfully copied, new actions can be introduced and only when these can be copied should the imitation of speech be attempted. The major problem presented by the teaching of speech is the lack of possiblities for using physical prompts, which makes imitation even more crucial for the development of these skills. Giangreco (1982) has suggested that by teaching imitation through functional tasks, multiplicity of purpose in teaching programmes can be increased.

Maintenance and Generalisation. In the field of applied behaviour analysis in general, and in its application to the field of mental retardation in particular, the issue of generalisation of learned behaviour has from the outset been a central concern. Many readers will be familiar with what has almost become an axiom in this area derived from Baer, Wolf and Risley's (1968) paper in Volume 1 of the *Journal of Applied Behavior Analysis*: 'In general, generalization should be programmed, rather than expected or lamented' (p. 97).

Yet despite this clear awareness of the problem, Stokes and Baer's (1977) later review in the same journal shows that remarkably little progress had been made in developing a technology that would ensure, or at least increase, the probability of taught behaviour generalising. In part, they attribute this to a theoretical view suggesting that generalisation was an essentially passive phenomenon: 'Something that happened, not something produced by procedures specific to it' (p. 349). These authors emphasise the importance of programming for generalisation and describe what they call an 'implicit embryonic technology'.

Stokes and Baer consider generalisation to be: '. . . the occurrence of relevant behavior under different, non-training conditions (i.e., across subjects, settings, people, behaviors, and/or time) without scheduling of the same events in those conditions as had been scheduled in the training conditions' (p. 350). They adopt what they call a 'pragmatic' approach to the issue of generalisation. They see it as occurring where no extra training manipulations are needed for extra training changes, or where if such extra manipulations are needed, their cost or extent is clearly less than that involved in the direct intervention.

If we preclude maintenance over time and interventions involving extra training manipulations of equal or higher cost than the original intervention, we are left with seven categories of *programmed* generalisation suggested by these authors. These were derived from the literature in the pragmatic spirit of their approach, rather than being based on *a priori* theoretical considerations. They are:

(i) Introduction to Natural Maintaining Contingencies: according to Stokes and Baer: '. . . the most dependable of all generalisation programming mechanisms', (p. 353). Here behaviours are chosen which will be likely to be naturally maintained in the wider ecology of the trainee.

(ii) Training Sufficient Exemplars: here sufficient (but not all) exemplars are trained to ensure that nontrained stimulus conditions and response conditions will occur.

(iii) Loose Training: here an attempt is made to teach under conditions in which there is considerable variation in both stimuli and responses. Relevant dimensions are therefore sampled enhancing the probability of generalisation in contrast to the more restricted conditions under which training typically takes place.

(iv) Use of Indiscriminable Contingencies: this is conceived of as an analogue to intermittent reinforcement with its well-documented effect of maintaining behaviour over time after withdrawal of reinforcement, more effectively than continuous reinforcement does. The parallel is that when a trainee cannot discriminate in which setting a response will or will not be reinforced, it is more likely to be generalised to other settings.

(v) Programming of Common Stimuli: here stimuli salient for the trainee are presented in both the training and generalisation settings.

(vi) Mediated Generalisation: Stokes and Baer identify mediation primarily with verbal mediation, though nonverbal mediation is by now a well-established process. The place of mediation in teaching self-management and self-control is noted.

(vii) Training to Generalise: here a generalised response can in itself be regarded as a reinforcible operant and examples of generalisation are reinforced with a view to establishing a class of generalised response wider than in the initial training repertoire.

In the conclusion to their paper, Stokes and Baer emphasise again the pragmatic nature of their approach, as well as suggesting specific applied techniques that should be brought to the attention of all those undertaking education and training with people with mental retardation.

Errorless Learning. Providing the individual with examples which are consistent with only one possible solution is argued to be most effective since it maximises opportunities for rewards to be given and teaching thus becomes a very positive and encouraging activity for pupil and teacher. Cullen (1976) and Engelmann (1977) provide examples of this technique known as errorless learning or errorless discrimination learning, the latter term reflecting the focus of its use on discrimination tasks. The task is gradually made more difficult by increasing the number of choice items or increasing the degree of difficulty of discrimination between distractors.

Cullen describes an example of applying these techniques to teach colour recognition to an individual using colour sample charts from a paint shop. The individual is presented with a bright red card only and asked to 'point to red'. Prompts are used and every response rewarded. When the individual is reliably pointing to the red card, a second card is introduced, perhaps being very pale yellow. Gradually the other colours are faded in and made brighter and brighter until the individual is able to point to red with salient distractors present. Sessions are then repeated using objects until the teacher is satisfied that the individual can reliably point to red. The procedure is then begun again with a second colour. This technique appears to be powerful especially for discrimination-type tasks and rewarding for both teacher and pupil.

Recording. The importance of recording is emphasised in many published curricula (see for example the Portage and Bereweeke materials reviewed later in this chapter) and it is likely that many teaching programmes fail at this point. The best programmes may be unsuccessful without precise measurement of the individual's progress. Effective evaluation techniques are needed to determine when the individual should move to the next step or programme and without careful recording much time, energy and enthusiasm may be wasted.

Systematic recording may be regarded as even more important with people with profound learning difficulties as the progress they make may be slow and subtle. Thus, progress may pass unnoticed by staff or parents in daily contact with the person if careful records are not kept. Choice of recording systems depends on the information that is required and the willingness of those carrying out the programme to sustain their commitment to record. The simplest system is therefore usually likely to be the most effective.

Precision teaching is a measurement procedure which has been successfully used with children with multiple impairments (Merbler and Harley 1977). It is a system with five steps. First the teacher must identify a specific behaviour he or she wishes to increase, decrease or maintain, which must be observable, countable and cyclical (i.e. have a definite beginning and ending). The second step is to write an instructional objective and develop an intervention plan. Third the teacher must count and record the occurrence of the specific behaviour daily, and fourth calculate the rate of the behaviour and transfer this information to a graph. The final step involves evaluating the child's progress and modifying the instructional procedure if the child is not progressing at a satisfactory rate.

Merbler and Harley report two main disadvantages of using precision teaching with people with multiple impairments. The first problem encountered was the rate ceiling effect when a child with physical and visual difficulties had apparently mastered the skill but could not perform it at a high rate because of his or her specific impairments. In this case the child's chart would reveal little improvement despite considerable progress. This problem can be overcome either by defining objectives in such a way that reliance on physical or visual skills are minimised or by graphing deceleration of incorrect responses as well as acceleration of correct ones. The second disadvantage of the precision teaching model is a more general problem that applies to any recording system in any educational context, that is, the infringement on teachers' direct contact time made by increased data collection activities.

The advantages of precision teaching are mainly concerned with the continuous monitoring it provides. It is more sensitive to progress than standardised tests and minimises wastage of time on ineffective programmes. Some teachers find the graphic display very reinforcing and no doubt parents likewise find it so.

A comprehensive and useful guide to recording is provided by Haring (1977). This focuses specifically on people with severe and profound learning difficulties and includes checklists, percentages (correct responses out of possible opportunities), frequency (number of responses within a specific period), latency measures (delay between instruction and response), duration (amount of time for which the behaviour continues), and trials to criterion. Haring distinguishes between measurement, assessment and evaluation. Measurement is a dynamic record of behaviour which charts performance, its rate, quality or quantity over time, perferably daily. Assessment is the recording of an individual's performance at any one time to determine his or her 'status' in skills or knowledge. Evaluation is the recording of an entire sequence or programme after it has been completed in order to assess its effectiveness.

For example, if an individual was on a toileting programme, the measurement would refer to the daily recording charts, the assessment to his or her score on the toileting section of the checklist completed at regular intervals and the evaluation would be a recording of the instances the individual used the toilet appropriately elsewhere, at home, at weekends and so on after teaching was completed. This would therefore provide information on generalisation and maintenance of the skill taught.

Within the category Haring has referred to as measurement, there are still a number of different ways in which the information can be collected. The frequency, duration or quality of the behaviour can be recorded in numerical terms. One step can be recorded trial by trial or the whole sequence of steps noted on each attempt as in Figure 2.2.

Figure 2.2: Examples of Recording

Recording trial by trial

Name:	Peter
Date:	8.11.84
Target:	Peter will grasp the spoon

Trial	Response
1	
2	
3	
4	
5	

Recording the whole sequence

Name: Peter   Date: 8.11.84

STEPS	TRIAL 1	2	3	4
Picks up spoon				
Scoops food				
Lifts spoon to mouth				
Opens mouth				
Takes food off spoon				
Chews and swallows food				

Many useful examples of recording are provided in Bailey (1983), Gardner *et al.* (1983) and in the Portage Guide (Bluma, Shearer, Frohman and Hilliard 1976) and the Bereweeke skill teaching system (Mansell, Felce, Jenkins and Flight 1984). These systems all have examples of cumulative record forms which enable daily record sheets to be dispensed with once the crucial information has been transferred to a cumulative record. An example from Gardner *et al.* (1983) is given in Figure 2.3.

Figure 2.3: Cumulative Assessment and Record Form

	Baseline results	Baseline results	Baseline results	Being taught	Learned	Checked
CORE AREA Self-help						
COMPONENT Dressing						
TARGET Child can button shirt independently.						
CONDITIONS With buttons ½-inch diameter.						
CRITERION Six times out of 10 for five consecutive days.						
STEPS 1. Grasps button between thumb and forefinger of right hand.						
2. Grasps left side of shirt, holding buttonhole between thumb and forefinger of left hand.						
3. Pulls or slightly folds back left side of shirt.						
4. Places button against thumb and pushes button half-way through buttonhole.						
5. Releases shirt with left hand and grasps the button with left forefinger and thumb.						

Source: Gardner, J., Murphy, J. and Crawford, N. (1983), *The Skills Analysis Model*, British Institute of Mental Handicap, Kidderminster. Reproduced by kind permission of the publishers BIMH Publications.

Aspects of the Task Presentation and Teaching Environment

The way in which a task is presented and the environment in which teaching takes place will be likely to influence the effectiveness of teaching programmes. Bell and Richmond (1984) have demonstrated with profoundly handicapped adults that manipulating the antecedents by orientating their attention to the task was more effective in improving task performance than the choice of reward offered. The procedure described previously, in the example of teaching colour discrimination through errorless learning techniques, illustrates the usefulness of masking or limiting part of the materials.

Positioning of the individual to be taught and of the teacher may be a factor contributing to the outcome of the programme. It is obvious that the individual should be comfortable with maximum support and able to reach any materials involved but the position of the teacher is often given less attention. Traditionally, individual teaching with this population often occurred with the teacher positioned behind or to the side of the person being taught. While this may be useful for some feeding and a few other specific programmes, it has the disadvantage of making it difficult for the teacher to see whether the individual is attending to the task.

Physical positioning at times other than during structured individual sessions may have important implications for skill development. Landesman-Dwyer and Sackett (1978) have shown that regularly placing people with profound and multiple handicaps in an upright position leads to better head control and increases the range of activities available to them. They also noted that positioning these individuals in pairs so that they were touching one another increased their exploratory behaviour.

In addition to the position of people involved in a teaching session, consideration should be given to other environmental aspects such as lighting, temperature, texture of surrounding materials and colour. All these aspects are dealt with in detail by Sandhu and Hendriks-Jansen (1976) in their comprehensive and stimulating account of environmental design for handicapped children which focuses on people with profound and multiple impairments. These authors studied hospital and school environments and the book has many practical suggestions for general design, layout of materials and specific equipment.

Group or Individual Instruction. DuBose (1977) has argued that cluster teaching and group instruction are far more characteristic of daily life than individual teaching and are effective training environments. The advantages of group instruction are not only concerned with overcoming lack of teacher hours available, but more positively, relate to teaching individuals to interact with their peers and increasing the opportunities to learn from 'models'. This should not be seen as incompatible with some of the teaching techniques discussed above as each individual in the group would be expected to have a clearly defined target which would probably differ from any other individual's target in the group.

However, group instruction may be less effective for the lowest functioning individuals because of the sustained physical assistance that needs to be given. Westling, Ferrell and Swenson (1982) found that group instruction was less effective, in terms of objectives taught, than individual instruction for children who are profoundly mentally retarded. They argued that these children should receive individual instruction until their attention and imitation skills are sufficiently well learned for them to be able to utilise the opportunities provided by a group. Perhaps DuBose's position which recommends a balance of individual and group work may afford the best compromise. We had some experience of the benefits of this model with an integrated preschool group of children ranging from those with profound learning difficulties through to those who were developing normally in a classroom in which each child received both group and individual instruction daily (see Gunstone, Hogg, Sebba, Warner and Almond 1982 for a full description of this).

Room Management. Closely related to the relative merits and disadvantages of group instruction for people with profound and multiple impairments is the use of room management systems. This method of organisation of staff in hospital wards, training centres and schools was first operationalised and evaluated by Porterfield, Blunden and Blewitt (1980) in order systematically to increase levels of adaptive behaviour. It involves two or more staff working with a group of people in such a way that maximum engagement in activities by the client group is maintained. The staff have very clearly defined roles as in the example in Figure 2.4 enabling one member of staff to carry out uninterrupted individual work or to maintain an 'activity period' with a group of people working on individual tasks. Many varieties of systems are used and in well staffed, tightly defined room management systems it might be possible to achieve and maintain both these activities simultaneously.

There are a number of examples of room management systems clearly increasing on-task behaviour of individuals and of the group as a whole (McBrien and Weightman 1980, Porterfield *et al.* 1980). Many of these examples involve people with profound and multiple impairments.

Figure 2.4: Example of Staff Roles in a Room Management Scheme

Room Manager/Activity Manager
1. Oversees all clients not in individual sessions.
2. Ensures each client has appropriate task.
3. Prompts unengaged clients, rewards engaged clients.
4. Moves from client to client quickly — only a few seconds with each one.
5. Does *NOT* toilet, mop up, leave room or deal with emergencies.

Mover
1. Toilets clients
2. Moves clients or equipment as requested by Room Manager.
3. Deals with all accidents, emergencies, visitors, etc.
4. When free, does individual work with client.

Individual Worker
1. Carries out short individual programmes with each client.
2. If Mover needs help, becomes second mover.

Source: Adapted from McBrien and Weightman (1980).

However, problems of maintenance are frequently noted (Coles and Blunden 1979) and it is important to stress that although a potentially powerful system, it is very demanding on staff and perhaps can only be carried out for short periods of the day.

Individualised Education Programme Plan. In the USA Public Law 94--142 mandates the development of a written Individualised Educational Plan (IEP) for every handicapped person. York and Williams (1977) outline the required content of the IEP which includes statements of the pupils present level of performance, the annual goals, the short-term objectives, the educational services required and the criteria and evaluation procedures to determine whether the goals and objectives are being achieved. This is not dissimilar to some of the requirements of the 'statements' introduced into England and Wales by the 1981 Education Act.

The Anson House Preschool Project (Gunstone *et al.* 1982) developed an individual programme plan format which specified the details of each teaching programme that was being taught with each child. It is shown in Figure 2.5 as an example of how programmes might be specified in order to ensure consistency, aid recording and enable other personnel to carry them out when the usual member of staff is unavailable. This plan is simple enough not to be too time-consuming to complete but does provide sufficient detail to enable continuity without confusion. Each individual might realistically have two or three of these programmes, one in each core area currently selected as a priority. Consolidation

Figure 2.5: The Individual Programme Plan

Target:
Task Analysis:
       (steps)
Rewards:
Prompts:
Presentation of Task
       Positioning:
       Special Materials:
       Instruction:
Structure of session
       Length of sessions:
       Time of Day:
Recording:
       Trial by trial, etc.

Source: Gunstone *et al.* (1982).

activities of an identical or related nature can be carried out during activity periods involving a room management scheme. Providing additional opportunities to practice skills has been demonstrated to increase acquisition of them (Lehr 1985).

Curriculum Resources

Resources consist mainly of staff and equipment. Before considering equipment there are two important points to be made concerning staffing. The first is that more staff does not necessarily result in higher levels of one-to-one teaching, since the more staff there are present, the more need there is for distinct roles and for consultation to take place between them. The strength of room management systems is that they attempt to ensure that staff interaction is minimised while maximising staff interaction with clients.

The second important point regarding staff is the recent trend in recognising that specialists such as physiotherapists, psychologists or speech therapists cannot provide a sustained clinical input to each individual client who requires it on a regular basis. For this reason models which involve transfer of skills from specialists to those in daily contact with the client group have become increasingly popular (see chapters by Warner and Almond in Gunstone *et al.* 1982). The physiotherapist, for example, has responsibility for several schools and a hospital clinic thus only enabling him or her to spend half a day a fortnight in a specific class for people with profound learning difficulties. Having initially assessed each client's needs and demonstrated a programme of management for each individual to the teacher, the therapist can use the fortnightly visits to supervise the teacher's execution of the recommended exercises and correct or clarify any difficulties that may have arisen.

Between the fortnightly visits the classroom staff can attempt to maintain a daily programme of exercises for each client.

Equipment. There are many examples of useful equipment for working with people with profound and multiple impairments and it is beyond the scope of this book to describe them all in detail. The reader is referred to Sandhu and Hendriks-Jansen (1976) or Simon (1981) for sources of some of these and to publications produced by physiotherapists, speech therapists and occupational therapists. Furthermore, there are many educational suppliers who now produce catalogues with specific sections on suitable equipment for this population. There has, however, been one area of development in this field which has dramatically expanded the opportunities for people with profound and multiple impairments. This is the area of microelectronics and, more specifically, microcomputers.

The development of applications of microelectronics with people with profound and multiple impairments has arisen from determined efforts to increase the opportunities for independence available to this population. As discussed in Chapter 3, this population lacks opportunities to exercise control over their environment. This arises from limited communication skills, restrictions on their ability to operate daily needs such as lights, radios, tape recorder, and a variety of toys. Related to this is the limited experience they have in order to develop understanding of cause and effect. Finally, the opportunities available to them for self-directed leisure activities are almost non-existent.

Most microelectronic equipment is based on a response-reinforcement model discussed in Chapter 3, which is central to the behavioural approaches. Many provide stronger and more varied sensory reinforcement than was ever previously available including sounds, moving pictures or objects, flashing lights, vibration and often combinations of two or more of these. Marlett (1984) describes these switch-controlled sensory reinforcers as perhaps the best example of a behavioural principle that has been used. She points out the need to vary both the switches and the sensory reinforcers to minimise satiation effects.

However, Byrne and Stevens (1980) have shown that careful selection of sensory stimuli should be made as children with multiple impairments were found to have marked variations in preference for visual or vibratory stimulation. The use of this type of stimulation to reduce stereotypies has also been reported in Murphy (1985) and is discussed again in Chapter 7 of this volume.

The input devices on microelectronic equipment are very varied. Pressure switches, in which variable pressure is required to operate them, can be activated by the hand, foot, head, arm, knee or shoulder. 'Joysticks' or levers are particularly useful with athetoid children and switches which operate by sucking or blowing through a tube are also very useful for those who have no use of limbs. The mercury switch was developed for those who can move arms or legs up or down but cannot exert any pressure. This switch is placed inside a band which can be attached to the arm or leg and is activated by moving the limb down and deactivated by moving it upwards. More information about switches and how to make them, microelectronic toys, communication aids and their use with people with profound and multiple impairments can be found in the Walsall Working Party (undated) curriculum, Rectory Paddock School (1983) curriculum and Woods and Parry (1981).

Microcomputers have likewise become increasingly popular in work with people with profound and multiple impairments. Similar arguments for their use apply as for the adapted toys described above. One of the clearest summaries of recent developments in the use of microcomputers with children with special educational needs is provided by Hogg (1984). Included in Hogg's booklet is the diagram which first appeared in a Schools Council (1982) publication showing the main applications of microcomputers to meeting special educational needs. These include their use as a planning aid, communication and mobility aid, electronic blackboard, reinforcer of basic skills, control device and very importantly to supply an individualised one-to-one approach. The most crucial but more general application given is the access microcomputers provide to the normal curriculum. It might be that for people with profound and multiple impairments the microcomputer offers access to the curriculum used by the rest of that Special School or facility. In short, as Behrmann and Lahm (1984) argue, computers will do many of the tasks that people with disabilities require other people to do for them today.

However, as Langford and Fidler (1983) point out there is some disparity between the actual and the proposed uses of microcomputers in education. Microcomputers can be programmed to provide individual targets at the student's level, pace the session according to the person's needs, tirelessly repeat lessons, and monitor progress by gathering, charting and analysing data. In order to do this in practice, additional hardware is often required because of the diversity of the individuals' goals. Microcomputer peripherals are not typically interchangeable and whichever model is chosen immediately restricts the software available.

Additional peripherals are being developed all the time. Concept keyboards enabling any overlay to be used instead of the ordinary keyboard, are particularly popular for work with people with profound and multiple impairments. They can be used, for example, to teach an individual the order in which items of clothing are put on. The program would produce an undressed figure on the screen and an overlay on the concept keyboard might show pictures of pants, vests, socks, shirt, trousers, jumper and shoes. If the order is important, for example, pants before trousers, the individual must touch the pants on the keyboard which will result in them appearing on the person on the screen. If the individual touches the trousers on the keyboard first, nothing happens. Many other similar programs involving everyday living skills exist. It is not suggested that these skills should be taught primarily on the microcomputer as this would essentially constitute teaching out of context. However, if for example, dressing is taught every morning when the person gets up, the microcomputer can be used to practice the skill and possibly build in generalisation. The software available for use with the concept keyboard appears to be more pedagogically appropriate than many of the programs generally available, probably because it has so far been produced mainly by teachers working with people with severe and profound impairments themselves.

Another important peripheral is the micromike. This is a microphone attachment which plugs into the microcomputer and can be used to encourage communication skills. The software which accompanies it includes drawing, colouring and other graphics which are operated by sounds made into the microphone. As yet, developments have not been sophisticated enough to enable graphics to respond to a single sound only at the exclusion of other sounds. This type of development is of great interest to speech therapists as well as teachers. Other uses of the microcomputer as a communication aid include the developments with speech chips which are enabling 'computer voices' to say what is being typed on the keyboard, and keyboard overlays which utilise whichever augmentative system is used by that individual, for example, a manual sign system, pictorial system or even Braille.

Microcomputers are providing a useful learning aid for people with multiple handicaps. Blenkhorn and Tobin (1984) report on their use with less able deaf-blind people, pointing out that light from a computer screen is emitted (as in a light bulb) rather than reflected (as from paper) which makes it particularly useful with people with only limited residual vision. The options offered by the microcomputer such as foreground and background colour, speed of movement and size of display provide more versatility, in terms of task presentation, for people with visual problems, than can usually be provided in the classroom. Stepp and Reiners (1983) report on a national conference in the USA on computer-assisted research and instruction for the hearing impaired which included applications to teaching speech, sign language, evaluating educational interventions and teacher training.

It is clearly important not to lose sight of our educational objectives by becoming drowned in technology. We need to ask ourselves regularly what the microcomputer is providing that could not be achieved without it. The answer to this question in relation to people with profound and multiple impairments at this time seems to be a great deal. They have access to the curriculum not previously possible, since any of the adapted switches described previously can be used to operate the software. They have opportunities to interact with others through educational or recreational activities on the microcomputer. If drill and practice is required, it can be provided endlessly with continuous monitoring of the child's responses. Reinforcement can be provided systematically and consistently although beware of programs which 'punish' incorrect responses with supposedly negative sounds or frowning faces, as many individuals find these equally or even more reinforcing than the intentional rewards. Ultimately the microcomputer may enable people with profound and multiple impairments to participate in educational activities on an individualised basis in a way which has previously been impossible given the resources available.

Sources of the Curriculum

Many schools and facilities prefer to develop their own curriculum using published ones as guides and selecting from each what appears most closely to meet their needs. This exercise of curriculum development and review may, as Hegarty *et al.* (1982) point out, be a useful process of in-service training involving staff in teamwork and advancing their skills. Through participating in the development, adoption, implementation, evaluation and refinement of the curriculum, teachers may learn about the different areas of development and how to devise, implement, evaluate and adapt instructional programmes (Williams and Gotts 1977).

In this section we will review the available published curricular materials in relation to the criteria that we consider relevant to staff working with people with profound and multiple impairments. These criteria have evolved from the suggestions made by staff attending training workshops on the education of people with profound and multiple impairments provided by the British Institute of Mental Handicap. Each criterion will be explained briefly before the curricula are reviewed. The criteria are as follows:

The Philosophical Basis of the Curriculum Should be Acceptable to the Staff Expected to Use It

Marlett (1984) identified four philosophical approaches with people with severe and profound handicaps: the adaptive/remedial approach; the developmental approach; the behavioural approach; and the functional approach. The adaptive/remedial approach is based on a medical notion of providing a 'cure', modification or adaptation for a problem, having first identified the underlying deficit. This approach has emphasised motor problems, cognitive structure and sensory problems. The main disadvantage of this type of approach is that the central conditions inherent in severe and profound disabilities cannot usually be permanently altered. However, it is a useful approach to identifying and intervening on remediable deficits such as hearing and visual problems.

The developmental approach, at its simplest, has based curriculum objectives on the achievement of specific 'milestones' as they occur in the development of the nonhandicapped child. Such sequences have usually been derived from developmental tests supplemented by information from more detailed studies of child development and direct observation of the client's behaviour. The approach provides the order for instructional objectives and the educational aim is to ensure that the highest developmental objective possible is attained. In reality it is difficult to distinguish this application of the developmental approach from the kind of sequence generated by a behavioural, task analysis orientation in which the steps are determined logically. For example, both approaches would prescribe the learning of one-word utterances before two-word utterances and walking with support before walking independently.

A more sophisticated approach to informing intervention through the use of developmental information argues that the processes involved in producing development must also be taken into account. For example, the recent work reviewed in Volume 1, Chapter 3 concerning the prerequisites of language development have clear implications for language programmes. The basis of early language in social interaction and cognitive prerequisites lead to a different emphasis and approach to teaching language than would result from simply following a series of objectives related to milestones. While the latter leads us into programmes in which several parallel strands (social and cognitive) are being worked on simultaneously to produce a particular outcome, the former is merely sequential. In subsequent chapters we will describe this approach to developmental programming more fully with respect to cognitive, communicative and motor development.

The behavioural approach employs a methodology in which specific intervention procedures are related to specific outcomes. Many of the techniques discussed earlier in this chapter such as setting objectives, task analysis, prompting, reinforcing and programming generalisation provide the foundation for the approach. The setting of objectives is undertaken with respect to an individual's current behaviour, in relation to a given curriculum. As noted above, such a curriculum may be similar to a developmentally derived curriculum, and in reality the curriculum designer may have drawn on developmental information.

The fourth approach that Marlett identifies, she refers to as the functional or future environments approach. This could be regarded as closely aligned to normalisation principles and in some ways represents an extension of the daily living and vocational skills within the behavioural approach. The work environment is used to teach vocational skills, the community environment used to teach recreation and self-help skills, and so on. The major shift in emphasis from the behavioural approach seems to be that the functional approach never removes the individual from his or her 'natural' environment in order to teach him or her a skill more intensively. It could be argued that behavioural approaches are being applied in an increasingly functional manner. The main disadvantage of this approach with people with profound and multiple impairments would seem to be that it assumes both physical and social integration. While this is philosophically a position for which we may strive, it is not at present an accurate description of the lives of most people with profound and multiple impairments.

Consideration of curricular materials therefore involves identification of the philosophical basis of the materials to see whether it is in keeping with the approach adopted by the relevant centre or school.

The Curricular Materials Should Cover Basic Skills Applicable to Clients with Very Low Skill Levels

The most frequent complaint made by staff attending training workshops is that materials start at skill levels which are too advanced for their clients. For example, the gross motor area starts with sitting, standing or walking skills when many of their clients have little or no head control, or the self-help skills start with eating with a spoon, whereas their clients cannot chew or swallow properly. We clearly need curricular materials aimed at teaching the most basic skills. However, as noted in Volume 1, Chapter 1, many clients in 'special care' units in schools or hospitals in England are not necessarily profoundly retarded but have marked additional impairments and severe behaviour disorders. Hence our curricular materials must also span the range applicable to people with severe learning difficulties.

The Curriculum Should be Capable of Dealing with a Variety of Sensory and Physical Deficits

In Volume 1, Chapter 1 we discussed the prevalence of additional impairments in people with profound learning difficulties. The very high prevalence noted of additional physical and sensory deficits suggests the need for curricular materials which offer adaptations that enable them to be used with clients with multiple impairments. Hence some suggestions on auditory and visual work to assist in the development of any residual hearing or vision are important. Similarly, detailed suggestions should be made of alternative physical positions or types of material to be used to take account of varying physical difficulties. Communication, which clearly warrants inclusion in every curriculum, should refer also to activities involving alternatives to speech such as the use of signing and symbol systems (see Chapter 4 of this volume).

The Curriculum Should Cover Sufficient Scope in Terms of its Core Areas and Components

It is useful to have all the main areas of the curriculum that are required within one set of teaching materials. It is harder work if the member of staff must refer to several different sources in order to cover all the core areas required. This is not to suggest that in developing a curriculum within a school or facility the staff should only use one source. Instead, the point to note is that particularly for untrained staff, it might be less overwhelming to be able to provide one consistent set of teaching materials which covers all the skill areas required. As a minimum, for people with profound and multiple impairments, these skill areas would seem to be cognitive skills, communication, motor competence and self-help skills.

The Curriculum Should State Clear Targets and Teaching Plans which Relate to Them

We are distinguishing between criterion-referenced checklists as discussed in Chapter 1 and curricular materials which may include a checklist but should also include suggested activities for teaching each of the skills that are listed. Targets, whether included as part of an assessment or as suggested teaching activities, should be clearly stated, leaving no question as to whether or not the client has achieved them. Teaching plans should state activities clearly, relate to each target and suggest methods of recording.

The Curricular Materials Should Contain Age-appropriate Items for Children and Adults or Make it Clear at which Population They Are Aimed

Most of the published curricula, as we shall see below, are aimed at staff working with children with profound and multiple impairments. The activities suggested often involve materials associated with young children and staff working with adults find it difficult to adapt the suggestions. Furthermore, motor skill activities suggested may be impossible for members of staff to carry out on their own with an immobile adult due to the size and weight of the client. Perhaps one of the reasons staff working with adults find this a particularly aggravating problem is because the resources for adults with profound and multiple impairments still lag behind those provided for children and there is still a paucity of written materials relating to adults.

The Cost of the Curriculum Materials should not preclude their Use and Where Possible Consumable Materials Required for Each Client such as Recording Sheets should be Reproducible.

This has been listed here as the last criterion but for the staff working with clients with profound and multiple impairments it is more likely to be at the top of the priority list on their criteria.

There are numerous curricular materials published in the UK, the USA and elsewhere in the world on teaching people with learning difficulties. Those relating to people with profound and multiple impairments are rarer. In reviewing these (see Table 2.1) we are aware that we have probably not covered everything that is available. Furthermore some of the material reviewed in Table 2.1 is not specifically for clients with profound and multiple impairments but has been used by staff who work with them and the applicability of such material may be of interest. We have used the seven criteria described above to give the reader a brief guide to what is available.

Holistic Approaches to Intervention

There has been much interest in methods of educating people with profound and multiple impairments which attempt to provide a total approach. Three of these holistic approaches, 'conductive education' ('Peto' after its originator), 'patterning' ('Doman-Delacato' after its originators) and 'co-active intervention' techniques will be briefly described. These have been selected as those most frequently used with people with profound or multiple impairments.

Conductive Education

Conductive education originated in Hungary where it was introduced by Peto and was brought to Britain by Esther Cotton, a physiotherapist, who introduced it to the Spastics Society. It is a holistic approach in which it is intended that the principles of conductive education are carried out throughout the day. It is a system designed for children with motor impairments, originally for those with normal intelligence but it has been applied in Britain and elsewhere to children with all levels of retardation. Jernqvist (1984), Rooke and Opel (1983), Cottam, McCartney and Cullen (1985) and Cottam and Sutton (1985) provide useful descriptions of this approach and Hegarty *et al.* (1982) describe a unit in which the curriculum is based upon it.

Conductive education makes no division between education and treatment, one person, the 'conductor', being the child's only teacher and carrying out the duties of therapists, care staff and teacher in all the child's functional daily skills. It is based on the theoretical work of Luria and other Soviet psychologists who believed that children can regulate their behaviour by verbalising their intentions, a process referred to as 'rhythmic intention'. For example, the conductor says: 'I will pick up my spoon' and the child repeats this (aloud or internally). The intention is then followed by the action.

These psychologists regarded verbal regulation in children with retardation as being ineffectively established due to the inadequate generalising function of their speech. Hence conductive education, which uses 'rhythmic intention' might be considered inappropriate for children who are unable to use speech in its regulatory function (Cottam *et al.* 1985).

Cottam *et al.* identify five major pedagogic aspects of conductive education: the conductor; group teaching; homogeneous groups; the philosophy that motor handicap can be overcome by teaching; and rhythmic intention. The conductor has already been mentioned. The group teaching is based on notions of collective discipline, competition and a concern on the part of each individual for the group's performance — not attributes noted among many of our 'special care' population. The conductive education groups should be homogeneous and physical handicap is regarded as a learning disability which can be overcome. Rhythmic intention has been described above.

The advantages of this approach appear to be the economy involved in a group programme, the cross-disciplinary approach which encompasses the child's total development. Furthermore, a functional approach

Table 2.1: Review of Published Curricula

Name	Reference	Brief Description of Contents	Philosophical Approach	Ability Level of Clients
Bereweeke Skill Teaching System	Mansell, Felce, Jenkins and Flight (1984)	Assessment checklist, Administrators' and Programme Writers' handbooks and record forms	Behavioural/ Functional	Moderate — Profound
Sensorimotor Cognitive Assessment and Curriculum for the Multihandicapped Child	Fieber (1977)	Adaptation of Uzgiris and Hunt (1975) Assessment of sensorimotor functioning with corresponding teaching suggestions	Developmental /Behavioural	Severe — Profound
The Skills Analysis Model	Gardner, Murphy and Crawford (1983)	Describes a six-stage curriculum model showing how to develop a core curriculum with detailed programme planning and recording; also chapters on staff training and parental involvement	Behavioural	Severe — Profound

Adaptations to Physical/ Sensory Handicaps	Scope — Areas Covered	Clear Targets and Teaching Plans	Age- Appropriate	Approx. Cost Reproducibility (1985)
None specifically given	Cognitive skills, perceptive and expressive language, self-care, gross motor social and practical skills	Targets clear, activity charts to be written by Programme Writer but handbook provided	Adults	Approx. £21, includes additional recording forms
Suggestions on positioning and adaptations for deaf/blind and visual impairments	Visual pursuit, localisation and object permanence, development of means for obtaining desired events, operational causality, motor imitation, vocal imitation, object relations in space and object schemes	Examples given in which targets, teaching plans and recording details are clearly stated	Children	Article in book
Not specifically	Social skills, communication, play and leisure, mobility and number	Numerous examples in each area of clear targets and teaching plans	Children	£6.00

Table 2.1: Cont.

Name	Reference	Brief Description of Contents	Philosophical Approach	Ability Level of Clients
A Comprehensive Program for Multi-handicapped Children	Jegard, Anderson, Glazer and Zaleski (1980)	Developmental checklist in each area followed by suggested activities — very simple and clear	Behavioural/ Developmental	Severe — profound
Analysis of Programmes for Teaching	Kiernan (1981)	Assessment lattices in each area followed by suggested teaching plans. Teaching techniques and recording are also covered	Behavioural	Severe — profound
A Prescriptive Behavioral Checklist for the Severely and Profoundly Retarded, Volumes I, II and III	Popovich (1977; 1981a and b)	Checklists with detailed objectives and teaching plans in three volumes, each representing more advanced skills	Behavioural	Severe — profound

Adaptations to Physical/ Sensory Handicaps	Scope — Areas Covered	Clear Targets and Teaching Plans	Age-Appropriate	Approx. Cost Reproducibility (1985)
All activities include suggestions for physical, auditory and visual impairments	Gross motor, fine motor, communication auditory, visual, tactile, olfactory and gustatory skills, body awareness	Each area has a number of objectives and teaching plans with useful illustrations	Children	£19.00
Suggestions for adapted activities	Teaching techniques and attention, social behaviour, co-operative play, choice, visual, sensorimotor, exploratory play, object permanence, delay and search strategies, discrimination, matching, shape, number, auditory, cause and effect	Each area has a number of clear targets and teaching plans with useful diagrams	Children	£6.95
Volume II specifically aimed at multiply impaired	Motor, eye-hand, language and self-help	The most comprehensive clear teaching targets and plans available e.g. five detailed programmes on head control	Children and school-leavers	£15.00 per volume

Table 2.1: Cont.

Name	Reference	Brief Description of Contents	Philosophical Approach	Ability Level of Clients
The Adaptive Behavior Curriculum Volume 1	Popovich and Laham (1981)	Checklists with each target task analysed. Written partly to provide basis for meeting requirements of Public Law 94–142	Developmental /Behavioural	Moderate – Profound
The Portage Guide to Early Education	Bluma, Shearer, Frohman and Hilliard (1976)	Manual explaining use of programme, checklist assessment colour coded according to area of development, and activity cards with teaching activities for each skill on checklist	Developmental /Behavioural	Mild – Severe
In Search of a Curriculum	Rectory Paddock School (1983)	A resource book giving teaching notes on wide range of areas of the curriculum with excellent pictures and examples of recording sheets. The appendices contain checklists of some of the areas covered and an extensive bibliography	Developmental /Behavioural	Moderate – Profound

Adaptations to Physical/ Sensory Handicaps	Scope — Areas Covered	Clear Targets and Teaching Plans	Age- Appropriate	Approx. Cost Reproducibility (1985)
None	Self-help, communication perceptual- motor, socialisation	Very clear targets and steps but no other details of programmes as such	Children and school- leavers	£16.00
None specifically given	Infant stimulation, self-help, motor, socialisation, cognitive and language	Targets not all clear. Teaching activities useful	Children	£57 whole kit. Additional checklists available
Chapter on multiple impairments	Cognitive, personal- social, language, reading, gross motor, housecraft, self-help, health education, religious education, creativity. Also chapters on parents, school-leavers, profound and multiple handicap	Clear objectives given in checklists in appendices. Teaching suggestions rather than plans in text	Children and school- leavers	£6.00

Table 2.1: Cont.

Name	Reference	Brief Description of Contents	Philosophical Approach	Ability Level of Clients
The Next Step on the Ladder: assessment and management of the multi-handicapped child	Simon (1981)	Book with checklist assessment at start of each chapter followed by illustrated training programme. Resource lists of equipment, further reading, etc.	Developmental /Behavioural	Profound
A Piagetian Approach to Curriculum Development for the Severely, Profoundly and Multiply Handicapped	Stephens (1977)	Article relating sensorimotor development to profoundly and multiply handicapped people. Has examples of appropriate teaching activities for items such as those in the Uzgiris and Hunt Assessment Scales (Uzgiris and Hunt 1975)	Developmental	Severe — Profound
Teaching the Multiply Handicapped	Walsall Education Department (undated)	Uses Gardner, Murphy and Crawford (1983) skills analysis model to give description of a curriculum for multiply handicapped	Behavioural	Profound

Adaptations to Physical/ Sensory Handicaps	Scope — Areas Covered	Clear Targets and Teaching Plans	Age-Appropriate	Approx. Cost Reproducibility (1985)
Suggestions for children with sensory/ physical impairments	Vision, auditory, gross and fine motor, social, self-help, communication (and signing)	Checklist targets reasonably clear. Teaching activities rather than plans	Children	£9.00
Specific suggestions for children with physical and/or sensory impairments	Sensori-motor, i.e. reflexive, primary, secondary and tertiary circular reactions, co-ordination of secondary schema, invention of new means. Also, pre-operational, i.e. preconceptual and intuitive	No targets given as such. Teaching suggestions for activities to develop at each stage	Children	Chapter in book
Suggestions throughout for those with sensory and/ or physical impairment	Self-help, mobility, stimulation, play, communication and environmental control	Examples of very clear targets and teaching plans in each area	Children	£2.00

Table 2.1: Cont.

Name	Reference	Brief Description of Contents	Philosophical Approach	Ability Level of Clients
		with chapters on each area and lots of illustrations of aids and equipment		
Curriculum Design for the Severely and Profoundly Handicapped	Wehman (1979)	In each skill area, reviews relevant research on attempts to teach severely and profoundly handicapped, and gives teaching suggestions with detailed examples. Also explains teaching techniques	Behavioural	Severe — Profound

Adaptations to Physical/ Sensory Handicaps	Scope — Areas Covered	Clear Targets and Teaching Plans	Age-Appropriate	Approx. Cost Reproducibility (1985)
A few suggestions for those with sensory and/ or physical impairments	Self-help, recreational skill development, vocational education, motor development, language, functional academics	Examples of very clear targets and teaching plans in each area	Children and Adults	£41.85

is implied in that daily living skills provide the content of the programme and positive attitudes of staff towards the programme clearly contribute to its value. However, in addition to the conductor extra staff are required to assist children's movements possibly up to staff level of 1:1. The need to carry out the programme so intensively may restrict other activities and the specialised equipment required, such as the ladder back chairs and plinths on tables, may raise resourcing problems.

The main disadvantage with conductive education appears to be the lack of empirical evidence suggesting it provides a more effective education than any of the other methods outlined in this chapter. Cottam *et al.* evaluated the effectiveness of this approach with children with profound learning difficulties by comparing it with other teaching methods and found no evidence of differences. This study is further considered in Chapter 5 of this volume.

Patterning

'Patterning' is a method popularised by Doman and Delacato (Doman 1974) at the Institute for the Achievement of Human Potential in Philadelphia. It has caused much controversy but is still popular with parents from all over the world who seek help for their brain-damaged children. The method originates in the work of an American neurosurgeon Temple Fay, who believed that the development of human movement followed a pattern which is predetermined biologically. The movements exhibited by the cerebral palsied child represented areas or levels of the brain which were undamaged. Emphasis was placed on pattern in human movement and it was seen as a task of the therapist to impose this pattern in the movements of people with cerebral palsy through exercises. Diet was also important to control intra-cranial pressure and the accumulation of spinal fluid.

In the 1950s, Doman, a physical therapist, set up a rehabilitation centre at which Fay was the consultant and Delacato an educational psychologist. The Doman-Delacato philosophy which developed argued that brain-damaged children should be given input through every sensory channel and encouraged to respond through motor functions. It also stated that the brain and body of the child should be in the best possible physical condition to maximise development. Robbins and Glass (1968) argued that the assumptions made by the Doman-Delacato philosophy are not supported by theoretical, experimental or logical scientific evidence.

The treatment recommended by the Institute involves eight to twelve hours a day, every day, usually requiring additional people to assist the parents, to enable them to do anything else, thereby turning the home into a public place. This has been one of the most controversial areas of the treatment since it is regarded as inhumane and liable to lead to family breakdowns. Doman argues that the intense activity provides relief for the family. Newman, McCann, Roos, Menolascino and Heal's (1977) survey of families involved in patterning programmes at home found little evidence of harmful effects on family relationships. Most studies have not focused specifically on these families but more generally on the effects of having a person with impairments in the family.

Studies of the effectiveness of the approach in terms of enhanced progress in the child, relative to that which might result from other approaches, are unclear. Newman, Roos, McCann, Menolascino and Laird (1974) found that children who were retarded and received patterning improved more on visual perception, programme-related measures of mobility and language ability than did the control groups (one of which received an alternative programme at the same intensity). However, intellectual functioning was not enhanced and Beasley and Hegarty (1976) describe some of the difficulties of using the programme-related measures provided by the Institute itself. These authors' own study on a British sample of children receiving patterning also found negligible changes in mental age but rather more significant gains in neurological age.

It is clear that the Doman-Delacato package offers something to parents that the statutory services are still not offering — an intensive programme of treatment in which parents are highly involved, plentiful relevant information (literature, etc. given out at the Institute), feedback on the results, equal partnership with professionals and ultimately hope. It is a clear statement on the lack of effective educational interventions being offered to families with children who have profound and multiple impairments, that they are willing to suffer financial hardship, emotional turmoil and sheer physical exhaustion to carry out a programme which still has little evidence to support it. It seems feasible to take a more eclectic approach and apply it comprehensively to prescribe a day-long programme which incorporates the usual daily routines rather than disrupting them.

Co-active Intervention Techniques

Co-active intervention techniques were initially developed for use with rubella-virus-damaged, deaf-blind children primarily by Van Dijk (1977), though the approach has subsequently been used with children who are retarded and physically impaired. It is based partly on the assumption that the foundation for all learning is initially motoric, and also on the fact that many deaf-blind children do have residual vision and hearing that they can employ with appropriate intervention. It is also claimed that other sense modalities, notably touch and smell, can be brought into play in a complementary fashion. Marlett (1984) gives co-active intervention as an example of a curriculum based on a developmental approach.

As with behavioural techniques, stress is placed on the initial development of clear programme objectives. Complete curricula have been produced and in chapters on given curricular areas in the remainder of this book we will draw on one of these written by McInnes and Treffry (1982). In contrast to behavioural approaches, great emphasis is laid on emotional bonding between teacher or parent and the child in the early stages of intervention. McInnes and Treffry write:

Regardless of which type your multiply sensorily deprived child is, the first step is to make contact with him and to begin to establish an emotional bond. You will provide the motivation which will encourage the child to reach outside himself and to initiate interaction between himself and the environment. (p. 19)

Intervention begins with close physical contact between teacher and child, e.g. with both on the floor and the latter supine between the teacher's legs. Chosen actions are guided by the teacher and the following sequences of reactions by the child described: resists; tolerates; cooperates passively; enjoys; responds co-operatively; leads; imitates; initiates. This sequence parallels the development of imitation from co-active responding, through to co-operative responding, and finally reactive responding.

Imitation is regarded as an important psychological development in ensuring that the child is learning to react to the environment. Similarly, co-active intervention will encourage anticipation, also bringing the child more fully into contact with reality. Activities involving rhythm and repetition encourage awareness of temporal order. Again, an emphasis in co-active therapy on temporal order will enhance short term memory (STM) according to Van Dijk (1977), STM being poor in deaf-blind children. Development of an understanding of temporal order is also seen as critical to the development of communication which constitutes a major curriculum target area for co-active therapy.

In this volume, we describe the use of co-active therapy with people with profound retardation and multiple impairments in early cognitive development (Chapter 3, pp. 121–4), communication (Chapter 4, pp. 153–5), motor competence (Chapter 5, pp. 190–1), and self-help competence (Chapter 6, pp. 215–18, 223) on the basis of McInnes and

Treffry's (1982) curriculum.

It should be borne in mind that the effectiveness of the approach with this group has yet to be evaluated and that these authors themselves are concerned that 'proven extreme brain damage' (p. 6) may limit its effectiveness. However, given the special problems of people who are deaf-blind and profoundly retarded, the techniques of co-active intervention do offer an approach to their education which is consistent with the developmental framework described in this book, and in several respects is comparable with specific behavioural techniques such as prompting, shaping and imitation.

Conclusion

In this chapter we have considered what constitutes a curriculum for people with profound and multiple impairments. We have outlined some of the objectives of such a curriculum, and the elements of it in terms of content areas, teaching methods and strategies, resources and aspects of the teaching environment. The sources of curriculum development have been briefly described and a number of published materials reviewed. Finally we considered three examples of holistic approaches to intervention for people with multiple impairments. In the next four chapters we consider in more detail some of the specific areas of development in which intervention can occur.

References

Ainscow, M. and Tweddle, D.A. (1981) 'The Objective Approach: A Progress Report' in R. Taylor (ed.), *Ways and Means 2*, Globe, Basingstoke

Baer, D.M., Peterson, R.F. and Sherman, J.A. (1967) 'The Development of Imitation by Reinforcing Behavioural Similarity to a Model', *Journal of Experimental Analysis of Behavior, 10*, 405–16

Baer, D.M., Wolf, M.M. and Risley, T.R. (1968) 'Some Current Dimensions of Applied Behavior Analysis', *Journal of Applied Behavior Analysis, 1*, 91–7

Bailey, I.J. (1983) *Structuring a Curriculum for Profoundly Mentally Handicapped Children*, Jordanhill College of Education, Glasgow

Baker, M., Jupp, K., Myland, E. and Thurlow, O. (1981) 'A Suggested Curriculum for the Profoundly Handicapped Child', *Apex, 8*, 132

Beasley, N. and Hegarty, J. (1976) *Doman-Delacato Treatment: Methods and Results*, University of Keele, Stoke-on-Trent

Behrmann, M.M and Lahm, L. (1984) 'Babies and Robots: Technology to Assist Learning of Young Multiply Disabled Children', *Rehabilitation Literature, 45*, 194–201

Bell, J. and Richmond, G. (1984) 'Improving Profoundly Mentally Retarded Adult's Performance on a Position Discrimination', *American Journal of Mental Deficiency, 89,* 180–6

Blenkhorn, P. and Tobin, M. (1984) 'Using Computers with the Less Able Deaf-Blind', *Sense, 30,* 6

Bluma, S., Shearer, M., Frohman, A. and Hilliard, J. (1976) *The Portage Guide to Early Education,* Cooperative Educational Service, Wisconsin

Brennan, W.K. (1974) *Shaping the Education of Slow Learners,* Routledge and Kegan Paul, London

Byrne, D.J. and Stevens, C.P. (1980) 'Mentally Handicapped Children's Responses to Vibrotactile and Other Stimuli as Evidence for the Existence of a Sensory Hierarchy', *Apex, 8,* 96–8

California State Department of Education (1976) *Learning Steps: A Handbook for Persons Working with Deaf-Blind Children in Residential Settings,* California State Department of Education, Sacremento

Coles, E. and Blunden, R. (1979) 'Establishment and Maintenance of a Ward-Based Activity Period within a Mental Handicap Hospital', *Research Report No. 8,*Mental Handicap in Wales, Cardiff

Committee on Special Educational Needs (COSPEN) (1984) *Learning Together: Issues in Designing a School Curriculum for Pupils with Severe Mental Handicap,* Scottish Curriculum Development Service, Glasgow

Cottam, P., McCartney, E. and Cullen, C. (1985) 'The Effectiveness of Conductive Education Principles with Profoundly Retarded Multiply Handicapped Children', *British Journal of Disorders of Communication, 20,* 45–60

Cottam, P. and Sutton, A. (eds.) (1985) *Conductive Education: A System for Overcoming Motor Disorder,* Croom Helm, London, Sydney and Dover, N.H.

Crawford, N.B. (ed.) (1980) *Curriculum Planning for the ESN(S) Child,* British Institute of Mental Handicap, Kidderminister

Cullen, C. (1976) 'Errorless Learning with the Retarded', *Nursing Times,* 25 March, 45–7

Doman, G. (1974) *What to Do about your Brain-Injured Child,* Cape, London

DuBose, R. (1977) 'Evaluation and Instruction of Severely and Profoundly Handicapped' in J. Cronin (ed.), *The Severely and Profoundly Handicapped Child,* State Board of Education, Illinois

Engelmann, S.E. (1977) 'Sequencing Cognitive and Academic Tasks' in R.D. Kneedler and S.G. Tarrey (eds.), *Changing Perspectives in Special Education,* Merrill, Ohio

Fieber, N.M. (1977) 'Sensorimotor Cognitive Assessment and Curriculum for the Multihandicapped Child' in J. Cronin (ed.), *The Severely and Profoundly Handicapped Child,* State Board of Education, Illinois

Gardner, J., Murphy, J. and Crawford, N. (1983) *The Skills Analysis Model,* British Institute of Mental Handicap, Kidderminster

Giangreco, M.F. (1982) 'Teaching Imitation to a Profoundly Delayed Learner Through Functional Tasks', *Education and Training of the Mentally Retarded, 17,* 163–7

Gunstone, C., Hogg, J., Sebba, J., Warner, J. and Almond, S. (1982) *Classroom Provision and Organisation for Integrated Preschool Children,* Barnardo Publications Ltd, Barkingside

Halle, J. and Touchette, P. (1986) 'Delayed Prompting: A Method for Instructing

Children with Severe Language Handicaps' in J. Hogg and P. Mittler (eds.), *Staff Training and Mental Handicap,* Croom Helm, London

Haring, N.G. (1977) 'Measurement and Evaluation Procedures for Programming with the Severely and Profoundly Handicapped' in E. Sontag (ed.), *Educational Programming for the Severely and Profoundly Handicapped,* Council for Exceptional Children, Reston, Va.

Hegarty, S., Pocklington, K. and Bradley, J. (1982) *Recent Curriculum Development in Special Education,* Schools Council Programme 4, Longman, York

Hogg, B. (1984) *Microcomputers and Special Educational Needs: A Guide to Good Practice,* National Council for Special Education, Stratford upon Avon

Hogg, J. (1985) 'Abnormality, Learning and Development in Profoundly Intellectually Impaired People and the issue of Educability', Paper delivered to the British Psychological Society Annual Conference, Warwick

Hotte, R.A., Monroe, H.J., Philbrood, D.L. and Scarlata, R.W. (1984) 'Programming for Persons with Profound Mental Retardation: A Three Year Retrospective Study', *Mental Retardation, 22,* 75–8

Jeffree, D.M., McConkey, R. and Hewson, S. (1977) *Teaching the Handicapped Child,* Souvenir Press, London

Jegard, S., Anderson, L., Glazer, C. and Zaleski, W.A. (1980) *A Comprehensive Program for Multihandicapped Children: An Illustrated Approach,* Alvin Buckwold Centre, Saskatchewan

Jernqvist, L. (1984) 'Two Views of Conductive Education', *Disability Now,* August, 5

Kiernan, C. (1981) *Analysis of Programmes for Teaching,* Globe Education, Basingstoke

Kiernan, C., Jordan, R. and Saunders, C. (1978) *Starting Off,* Souvenir Press, London

Landesman-Dwyer, S. and Sackett, G.P. (1978) 'Behavioral Changes in Non Ambulatory Profoundly Mentally Retarded Individuals' in C.E. Meyers (ed.), *Quality of Life in Severely and Profoundly Mentally Retarded People: Research Foundations for Improvement,* American Association on Mental Deficiency, Washington, D.C.

Langford, C.A. and Fidler, P.S. (1983) 'Microcomputers for Severely Handicapped Students: Issues in Design and Evaluation', *American Annals of the Deaf, 128,* 605–9

Lehr, D. (1985) 'Effects of Opportunities to Practice on Learning Among Students with Severe Handicaps', *Education and Training of the Mentally Retarded, 20,* 268–74

McBrien, J. and Foxen, T. (1981) *Training Staff in Behavioural Methods: The EDY In-Service Course for Mental Handicap Practitioners,* Manchester University Press, Manchester

McBrien, J. and Weightman, J. (1980) 'The Effect of a Room Management Procedure on the Engagement of Profoundly Retarded Children', *British Journal of Mental Subnormality, 50,* 38–46

McInnes, J.M. and Treffry, J.A. (1982) *Deaf-Blind Infants and Children 'A Development Guide',* University of Toronto Press, Toronto Open University Press, Milton Keynes

McLean, E. (1984) 'Ward Teaching Won't Do!', *Child: Care, Health and Development, 10,* 261–71

Mansell, J., Felce, D., Jenkins, J. and Flight, C. (1984) *Bereweeke Skill-Teaching System,* NFER-Nelson, Windsor

Marlett, N. (1984) 'Program for the Severely and Profoundly Handicapped: The Last Educational Frontier', unpublished manuscript, Special Education Symposium, King Alfred's College, Winchester

Merbler, J.B. and Harley, R.K. (1977) 'Implementation of a Precision Teaching Data Collection System in a Program for Multiply Handicapped Visually Impaired Children', *Education of the Visually Handicapped, 8,* 97

Murphy, G. (1985), 'Self-Injurious Behaviour in the Mentally Handicapped: An Update', *Association for Child Psychology and Psychiatry Newsletter, 7,* 2–11

Murphy, R.J. and Doughty, N.R. (1977) 'Establishment of Controlled Arm Movements in Profoundly Retarded Students Using Response Contingent Vibratory Stimulation', *American Journal of Mental Deficiency, 82,* 212–16

Newman, R., McCann, B.M., Roos, P., Menolascino, F.J. and Heal, L.W. (1977) 'A Survey of Parents Using Sensorimotor Home Training Programs', *Education and Training of the Mentally Retarded, 12,* 109–18

Newman, R., Roos, P., McCann, B.M., Menolascino, F.J. and Laird, W.H. (1974) 'Experimental Evaluation of Sensorimotor Patterning Used with Mentally Retarded Children', *American Journal of Mental Deficiency, 79,* 372–84

Pace, G.M., Ivancic, M.T., Edwards, G.L., Iwata, B.A. and Page, T.J. (1985) 'Assessment of Stimulus Preference and Reinforcer Value with Profoundly Retarded Individuals', *Journal of Applied Behavior Analysis, 18,* 249–55

Perkins, E.A., Taylor, P.D. and Capie, A.C.M. (1980) *Helping the Retarded: A Systematic Behavioural Approach,* British Institute of Mental Handicap, Kidderminster

Popovich, D. (1977) *A Prescriptive Behavioral Checklist for the Severely and Profoundly Retarded: Volume I,* University Park Press, Baltimore

Popovich, D. (1981a) *A Prescriptive Behavioral Checklist for the Severely and Profoundly Retarded: Volume II,* University Park Press, Baltimore

Popovich, D. (1981b) *A Prescriptive Behavioral Checklist for the Severely and Profoundly Retarded: Volume III,* University Park Press, Baltimore

Popovich, D. and Laham, S.L. (1981) *The Adaptive Behavior Curriculum,* Paul H. Brookes Publishing Co., Baltimore

Porterfield, J., Blunden, R. and Blewitt, E. (1980) 'Improving Environments for Profoundly Handicapped Adults', *Behaviour Modification, 4,* 225–41

Presland, J.L. (1980) 'Educating "Special Care" Children: A Review of the Literature', *Educational Research, 23,* 20–33

Rectory Paddock School (1983) *In Search of a Curriculum,* Robin Wren Publications, Bromley

Remington, R.E., Foxen, T. and Hogg, J. (1977) 'Auditory Reinforcement in Profoundly Retarded Multiply Handicapped Children', *American Journal of Mental Deficiency, 82,* 299–304

Robbins, M.P. and Glass, G.V. (1968) 'The Doman-Delacato Rationale: A Critical Analysis' in J. Hellmuth (ed.), *Educational Therapy,* Special Child Publications, Seattle

Rooke, P. and Opel, P. (1983) 'An Approach to Teaching Profoundly Multiply Handicapped Children', *Mental Handicap, 11,* 73–4

Sandhu, J.S. and Hendriks-Jansen, H. (1976) *Environmental Design for*

Handicapped Children, Saxon House, Farnborough

Schools Council Report (1982) *Microcomputers in Special Education*, Longmans, London

Simon, G.B. (1981) *The Next Step on the Ladder*, British Institute of Mental Handicap, Kidderminster

Stainback, W. and Stainback, S. (1983) 'A Review of Research on the Educability of Profoundly Retarded Persons', *Education and Training of the Mentally Retarded, 18*, 90–100

Stephens, B. (1977) 'A Piagetian Approach to Curriculum Development for the Severely, Profoundly and Multiply Handicapped' in E. Sontag (ed.), *Educational Programming for the Severely and Profoundly Handicapped*, Council for Exceptional Children, Reston, VA

Stepp, R.E. and Reiners, E. (1983) 'Computer Assisted Research and Instruction for the Hearing Impaired', *American Annals of the Deaf, 128*, 507–774

Stokes, T.F. and Baer, D.M. (1977) 'An Implicit Technology of Generalisation', *Journal of Applied Behavior Analysis, 10*, 349–67

Tansley, A.E. and Gulliford, R. (1960) *The Education of Slow Learning Children*, Routledge and Kegan Paul, London

Uzgiris, I.C. and Hunt, J.McV. (1975) *Assessment in Infancy. Ordinal Scales of Psychological Development*. University of Illinois Press, Urbana

Van Dijk, J. (1977) 'What We Have Learned in 12½ Years: Principles of Deaf-Blind Education' in M. Jurgens (ed.), *Confrontation Between the Young Deaf-Blind and the Outer World*, Swets and Zeitlinger, Lisse

Walsall Working Party (undated) *Teaching the Multiply Handicapped*, Walsall Education Department, Walsall

Wehman, P. (1979) *Curriculum Design for the Severely and Profoundly Handicapped*, Human Sciences Press, New York

Westling, D.L., Ferrell, K. and Swenson, K. (1982) 'Intraclassroom Comparison of Two Arrangements for Teaching Profoundly Mentally Retarded Children', *American Journal of Mental Deficiency, 86*, 601–8

Williams, W., and Gotts, E.A. (1977) 'Selected Considerations on Developing Curriculum for Severely Handicapped Students' in E. Sontag (ed.), *Educational Programming for the Severely and Profoundly Handicapped*, Council for Exceptional Children, Reston, V.A.

Wilson, M.D. (1981) *The Curriculum in Special Schools*, Schools Council, London

Woods, P. and Parry, R. (1981) 'Pethna: Tailor-Made Toys for the Severely Handicapped', *Apex, 9*, 53–6

York, R. and Williams, W. (1977) 'Curricula and Ongoing Assessment for Individualised Programming in the Classroom' in J. Cronin (ed.), *The Severely and Profoundly Handicapped Child*, State Board of Education, Illinois

3 DEVELOPING COGNITIVE ABILITIES

Sensorimotor Teaching

Though we have adopted a broadly based consideration of child development, we have emphasised the Piagetian account of early cognition, especially with reference to sensorimotor and preoperational development. Such an approach is facilitated by the recent development of assessment instruments that have been shown to be applicable to people who are profoundly retarded. In this chapter, the extension of the Piagetian analysis of early cognition to curriculum development is described. In introducing this subject we cannot improve on Stephens' (1977) own introduction to the topic of developing programmes in the light of Piaget's theory:

> A Piagetian approach to curriculum development is one that emphasises the process of learning, rather than the product. It is one that emphasises the need for the pupil to be actively involved in the learning situation; the need for him to proceed at his own tempo; and the need for him to explore and to manipulate, to question and to seek — in short, to learn to reason. What is sought is a comprehensive curriculum that extends horizontally, to provide the repetition or variety of experiences generally required by the severely and multiply handicapped for the mastery of a skill. Yet it must also extend vertically, through closely sequenced activities that are designed to lead the pupil, slight achievement by slight achievement, up the developmental scale. To date, there is not one program which has both sequentially related and branching activities plus the adaptations which are necessary if they are to be used with a variety of handicapped individuals (e.g. deaf-blind, cerebral palsied-mentally retarded, etc.). Therefore the programmer will of necessity draw from a variety of existing resources, identify lacunae, and then set about adapting or devising individually appropriate activities. As one proceeds it is evident, at the sensory-motor and pre-operational levels, activities labelled 'motor' or 'social' also include elements of reasoning or cognitive development. (p. 247)

The position described by Stephens still holds and raises the questions as to how best to approach the organisation of available material. On the one hand, it is possible to present programme suggestions and illustrations in terms of the main categories of schema development during the sensorimotor period. We would here focus on schema in the Reflexive period and those of Primary Circular Reactions, Secondary Circular Reactions, Co-ordination of Secondary Schema, Tertiary Circular Reactions and Invention of New Means through Mental Combinations. On the other hand, we could focus concern on the domains defined in an assessment procedure of the kind described by Uzgiris and Hunt (1975) or Dunst (1980). Thus we would consider: The Development of Visual Pursuit and the Permanence of Objects; The Development of Means for Obtaining Desired Environmental Events; Imitation; The Development of Operational Causality; The Construction of Object Relations in Space; and The Development of Schemes for Relating to Objects. In the event, we are going to opt for a combination of these approaches. With respect to sensorimotor development, early behaviour is relatively undifferentiated. With development come the increasingly distinguishable domains listed above. It therefore seems reasonable to begin by considering the enhancement of the basic activities and schemes exhibited in the first three sensorimotor stages, the Reflexive and the Primary and Secondary Circular Reaction stages. We will then deal with the curriculum in terms of the main areas of development through Stages III–VI and into critical activities in the intuitive phase of the preoperational stage.

Having said which, we must emphasise another point made by Stephens, namely that any given piece of behaviour reflects not only motor, social and cognitive aspects, but also in any one task a variety of cognitive components. Thus, the ability to retreive an invisible object with a stick, for example, a ball that has rolled under the chair, reflects both object permanence and means-end behaviour — as well as the ability to adopt an appropriate grasp and the motivation to continue the social activity of playing with another person. Any opportunity to teach a specific skill is therefore an opportunity to deal with a variety of other important experiences and events.

Finally, Stephen's claim that we do not have a comprehensive curriculum for people who are profoundly retarded and multiply impaired also still holds good. In what follows, then, we range from highly specific approaches often derived from experimental studies to more general suggestions on developmentally suitable activities. Following these reviews, we relate some aspects of this emerging curriculum to the needs of those with multiple sensory impairments, in addition to mental retardation.

Developing Cognition in Sensorimotor Stages I, II and III

Many profoundly retarded people will be functioning in Piaget's Reflexive and Primary and Secondary Circular Reaction Stages. It is highly likely that this will reflect extensive impairments to the central nervous system affecting both motor and sensory systems. Much of what will need to be done will therefore be at a therapeutic level of intervention, the physiotherapist and the speech therapist encouraging normal reflex development and sensitising or desensitising responsiveness in the various modalities. Approaches in these areas will be discussed in subsequent chapters. Success here will not only have remedial benefits in its own right, but will lead to improvements in cognition that open up the way for future work on sensory development.

As explained in Chapter 3 in Volume 1, Piaget's view of reflexive behaviour should not be taken as a strictly neurological one. He is more concerned to describe the entire repertoire of behaviours the newborn child has at its disposal and their co-ordination during the first months of life. Stephens (1977) and Fieber (1977) have described the development of the curriculum in this period, Stephens for severely and profoundly retarded people in general, Fieber for multiply handicapped children in particular. For both, intervention centres on the development of grasp, sucking and vision.

Grasp. Stephens emphasises the importance of the development of grasp in Stage I. She suggests that palmar grasp can be improved by placing the teacher's finger or a long object (a dowel or rattle handle) in the child's hand and tugging it in order to strengthen the grasp. If the child's grasp is too weak, then the teacher should place his or her hand around it and mould the grip. As the grip increases, so this support would be faded. The resulting ability to hold is in fact the first item to be recorded on Uzgiris and Hunt's Scale VI: The development of schemes for relating to objects, an item split into 'Grasps examiner's finger' (E48) and 'Retention of objects' (E49) by Dunst. As we saw in Chapter 3 of Volume 1, the development of grasp evolves as the palmar reflex disappears. Voluntary grasping will initially be directed to clothing and objects with which the hand comes into contact. As Fieber (1977) notes, children with tightly fisted hands, abnormal postures and restricted movement may not encounter objects in this way, a fact that emphasises the need for the teacher to place objects in the hand in the manner described above. Fieber also suggests how this activity can be dealt with in a formal behavioural fashion, timing the duration of grasping on five or six trials following active intervention and prompting. Such an approach also implies that a behavioural target of success has been set, e.g. hold object for 15 seconds plus on five out of six trials.

Sucking. We have seen the importance Piaget places on the infant's sucking of objects. Stephens suggests encouragement of the rooting behaviour by tickling the infant's face near the mouth, then transferring stimulation to the other side when the head turns. Fieber (1977) points out that operant sucking, i.e. sucking for a reinforcer, whether food or some sensory experience, has been demonstrated with nonhandicapped, newborn infants. The possibility of developing sucking operantly with both food or some other object might be a valuable adjunct to the stimulation techniques noted.

Visual Tracking. The Uzgiris-Hunt Scale 1: The Development of Visual Pursuit and the Permanence of Objects has only one visual tracking item, namely: follows a slowly moving object through an arc of 180°. Stephens and Fieber advocate the development of programmes to teach or encourage such tracking. However, while it is appropriate to begin with horizontal tracking of the sort recorded on this item of the Uzgiris-Hunt Scales, it is important to bear in mind that more developmentally advanced tracking in the vertical plane and also circular tracking would subsequently need to be attempted. Note, too, the conditions described in an assessment of this sort ('Hold object about ten inches in front of the infant's eyes, until he focusses on it', Uzgiris and Hunt 1975, p. 151). Using a soundless multi-coloured object might well require modification. For children with visual impairment or who might be expected to be inattentive to such an object, a bright light source would be more appropriate and this might need to be presented in a darkened room. In addition, for remedial purposes, a sound could accompany movement of the object during the early stages of the programme though this would be faded and eliminated as the child came to attend to visual cues. The direction to ensure that the child is focusing on the object at the start of the trajectory is, of course, essential.

Taken together these factors would be reflected in baseline assessments as Fieber suggests, i.e. with respect to (i) arc; (ii) eye movement vs eye-head movements; (iii) direction; and (iv) the characteristics of the object to be tracked, i.e. brightness, size, speed, etc. To these we might add (v) the setting in which the object is presented, i.e. level of room illumination, plainness of background, other distractors, etc.

Other Bodily Movements. Though Piaget concentrates mainly on the hand, it is clear that other parts of the child's body can become engaged in schema-like activity. Stephens emphasises encouragement of kicking and arm waving. However, we can offer response opportunities to people who are multiply impaired and with gross physical difficulties involving any part of the body they can move. Hogg (1983), for example, socially and visually reinforced a head turn from mid-line to the right in a boy who was profoundly retarded and for whom this was the only available gross motor action. (A full description of this appears in Chapter 9 of Volume 1).

In parallel to the co-ordination of schemes is the development of Primary Circular Reactions. Brinker and Lewis (1982b) nicely capture the distinction between Primary and Secondary Circular Reactions in the following description as if from the infant's point of view:

> Primary Circular Reaction — I can make things happen (but I don't know how I did it)
> Secondary Circular Reactions — I can make this response to make this event happen

The development of such Circular Reactions in infants has been referred to as 'contingency analysis' or 'contingency learning'. While Piaget distinguishes the two stages *as* stages, in reality we are likely to see a child becoming frequently proficient in learning to act upon his or her environment and the progression suggested by Brinker and Lewis will tend to reflect a continuum rather than a distinct break noted in qualitatively different types of behaviour. Brinker and Lewis (1982a, b) do suggest two ways in which a distinction between primary and secondary circular actions can be drawn. With respect to Primary Reactions, generalised body or limb movements will be observed to produce the contingency. More discrete actions, e.g. an arm movement, will eventually develop, indicative of Secondary Reactions. If this differentiation is maintained across sessions, then Secondary Reactions may be considered to be established. Where, however, relearning of the discrete action has to take place in each session, the person may be regarded as being basically at the Primary stage. It is interesting to note that virtually all reports of operant learning in people who are profoundly retarded and multiply impaired indicate that a refining of general bodily movement into discrete action does take place.

With respect to Uzgiris and Hunt's Scales, items relevant to Primary and Secondary Circular Reaction occur on both Scale II: The Development of Means for Obtaining Desired Environmental Events and Scale

IV: The Development of Operational Causality. With respect to the former, in situation 3, a pass is awarded for the Secondary Circular Reaction 'Repeats arm movements systematically and keeps toy active consistently' (Dunst scale step 2 on this scale). In the latter we find situation 2 in which activation of a toy is again scored, plus situation 3c where the child employs 'A dominant act during pauses suggesting a procedure'. Both items appear on the relevant scales in Dunst.

In the literature concerned with people who are profoundly retarded and multiply impaired, the development of Primary and Secondary Circular Reactions has been approached through recommendations on (i) the type of play or activities that will enduce the association between action and outcome that characterises these behaviours; (ii) through direct operant training; and (iii) through what has been called contingency interventions.

With regard to the first of these, suggested play activities, Stephens recommends simple integrated activities such as attaching a floating toy to a child's wrist by a piece of string while the child is in a pool. Naturally occurring movements will lead to the toy bobbing in the water and it is hoped that the child will repeat the activity even though the contingency is not necessarily clearly established. She regards this as essentially a Primary Circular Reaction situation, while her recommendation for encouraging Secondary Circular Reactions is more structured. Here the use of squeeze and squeak toys and others that produce a definite effect is recommended. A variety of commercially available toys are suitable for such activities, though adaptation to take into account the particular impairments of a given person may be required.

Easy though it is to suggest situations and toys in which Circular Reactions can be encouraged, it is essential we get away from any simple notion that exposure to such situations will 'stimulate' the person's development. We are actually trying to establish a very complex link between the person's own behaviour and an outcome. For that reason the means by which the person effects the outcome must be carefully devised to ensure that a response is available within the motor repertoire and that the visual, auditory or movement consequence can be clearly determined by the person.

We have already described in some detail the first, experimental, operant approaches to teaching Circular Reactions to profoundly retarded multiply impaired people in Chapter 9 of Volume 1. The work of Fuller (1949), Piper and MacKinnon (1969) and Rice and his colleagues illustrate the way in which specific behaviours within the individual's repertoire can be shaped using a variety of reinforcers. The reinforcers, as we noted, ranged from basic biological reinforcement such as food to a variety of sensory events, visual, auditory and vibratory. The starting point for programme development is reflected in much of this work, particularly that of Rice. Decisions must be made regarding available responses that the person who is profoundly retarded and multiply impaired might make in order to produce a consequence, while effective reinforcers must also be established, with respect to actions possible in upper and lower limb movement, trunk and head control. Where a particular movement appears to be under high reinforcement control, as in the case of hand waving or eye poking, the reinforceability of alternative movements would also have to be taken into account. In addition, the positioning of the person to permit execution of their chosen movement would have to be determined. As we have seen in Chapter 9 of Volume 1, the selection of reinforcers is a matter of both observation and experience of the person, as well as trial and error. It should be added that any information we have on sensory abilities of the individual will also enter into our consideration of potential reinforcers.

While we are emphasising in this account of programme development the teaching of specific behaviours that will have adaptive value, it is also important to note some wider motivational aims. Brinker and Lewis (1982c) emphasise that motor or intellectual impairment can lead a child to experience the world as essentially uncontrollable, resulting in declining motivation to attempt to exercise direct control. They suggest that the learning of such helplessness can affect both their individual experience of the physical world and social interactions. We have already seen the interdependence of early interactions and the development of communication and Brinker and Lewis rightly comment that 'reduction in social contingencies disrupts the very cradle of meaning and has effects on the further development of both language and thought' (p. 164).

The general information on our approach to teaching Circular Reactions can be illustrated through a flow chart developed to direct the studies in this area carried out by Remington, Foxen and Hogg (1977). Figure 3.1 is adapted from Remington (1975) and shows the decisions that would have to be taken in order to develop and monitor such a programme.

Note, first, that our concern is not initially to teach an obvious, adaptively useful action. In line with Brinker and Lewis, the intention is to give the person the opportunity to exercise control over his or her environment and for that reason any available movement might be selected. The first box in the flow chart in Figure 3.1, therefore, suggests that we take a baseline on the selected action (1). If we find that this occurs at a low level, i.e. only on a few occasions during the period that we propose to carry out our teaching sessions (e.g. 5, 10, 15 minutes) then we would proceed with the programme, i.e. if we answer 'yes' to the question 'Person has low operant level?' (2) we proceed. If the level is already high and the answer is 'no', then we would look for an alternative action.

On the basis of our observations we would select a reinforcer and make this available when the action occurs (3). If, however, it does not occur spontaneously (4), then we would begin to prompt and shape the action (4a). If this is successful, then we would continue reinforcing the taught action just as we would had it occurred spontaneously without our direct intervention (5). Failure after our intervention would lead us to change our reinforcer to another that might be potentially reinforcing (4c). Success here would return us to (3) and we would re-embark on our cycle. If the diagram is again followed then it will be seen that several cycles through (4)-(4a)-(4b)-(4c) may be attempted before the combination of teaching procedures and reinforcement prove effective. When spontaneous actions are demonstrated (4), then we would proceed with reinforcement (5) and establish if the action is maintained under condition (6). Should responding decline, then the person may be having too much of the reinforcer, i.e. satiating (6a). In response to this we would change the reinforcer (4c) and recommence the cycle from (3). If responding is maintained on FR1 then we introduce *partial* reinforcement which involves *not* reinforcing every time the target action occurs, e.g. randomly reinforcing only one out of two correct responses, or every other response (7). The actual ratio of reinforced to nonreinforced responses can be increased or stretched indefinitely though at some point it will cease to be effective and responding will decline and extinguish. However, by introducing partial reinforcement and extending the ratio to some degree the person's motivation to work for the reinforcer can be increased. There are good reasons for introducing partial reinforcement. First, general operant theory and its application to people with mental handicap has shown that partial reinforcement leads to better maintenance of an action than does continuous reinforcement (Hogg 1975). Second, the approach to people who are profoundly retarded and multiply impaired that we are advocating is a highly structured and artificial one. The nonhandicapped infant making Circular Reactions does not confront a totally predictable world and much of the motivation to explore that world must come from the fact that the outcome of actions is not invariably predictable. Here, however, we are dealing with people with major learning difficulties and we can attempt to simulate the real world by introducing some measure of unpredictability. Even so, if on

Figure 3.1: Systematic Procedure for Establishing Circular Reactions Through Operant Techniques

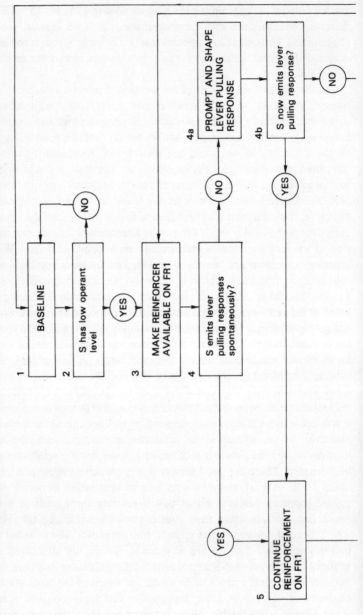

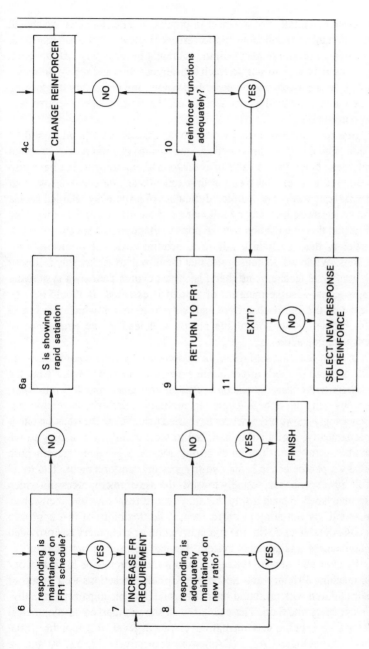

Source: Adapted from Remington (1975).

introducing partial reinforcement responding did decline, then we should have to return to continuous reinforcement as shown in (9). Alternatively, a change of reinforcement (10) to (4c) might be necessary. At this point (11), we may wish to start to teach a different action and we would return to (1). In approaches to be described below, the possibility of teaching a new action as well as, or instead of, the first chosen objective will be considered.

Before dealing with this work, however, a general point should be made. The flowchart presented and the various operations in it have not only been employed in carefully constructed experiments but have also been used to guide intervention in practical teaching situations without special equipment. The learning difficulties of profoundly retarded people can be so severe that only by following and recording a series of teaching aims and their realisation can we hope to diagnose the specific areas of difficulty that result in a failure to acquire basic early sensorimotor actions. While we do not suggest that the flowchart is slavishly followed — individual teachers and therapists must evolve their own systematic approaches — some measure of system is essential. It should also be clear that the approach differs markedly from that in which it is hoped that simple stimulation of the person will lead to the emergence of sensorimotor actions.

In many teaching settings the development of sensorimotor behaviours will proceed through direct interaction of teacher and pupil. Thus the teachers will observe the action, e.g. an arm raise, and will reinforce, e.g. by ringing a bell where an auditory reinforcer is employed. Increasingly, however, teachers have tried to automate the situation either mechanically, e.g. a string attached to the person's arm leading to the bell being rung, or through electronic means, e.g. where an arm raise breaks a photoelectric beam and triggers the reinforcement. The trend will, however, be increasingly towards the use of microprocessors which are interfaced in such a way that they record responses and themselves 'respond' by initiating reinforcement. The flexibility of this approach is considerable and with the miniaturisation of computers has provided a convenient and portable system that can be used in any setting.

Brinker and Lewis (1982a) utilised a microprocessor in their work on teaching Primary and Secondary Circular Reactions to a group of four children with profound retardation and multiple impairments, Sally, Tracy, Mary and Sian. These children all showed marked developmental delays, each being at a mental development level of 2 months whille their Chronological Ages (CAs) were respectively 29, 52, 40 and 40 months. Actions were selected for each child and appropriate reinforcers determined. By the use of simple devices that automatically registered a kick on a panel or lever pull a microcomputer automatically initiated a variety of reinforcing events, auditory, visual or tactile. If the response itself could not be automated, then the teacher would observe that action and press a button that would, via the computer, produce the chosen reinforcer.

Sally, a child damaged by cytomegalovirus and with spastic hypotonia and quadriplegia, was reinforced by the operation of a musical mechanised toy for two actions — an arm movement and leg kicking. Tracy, microcephalic and with spastic hypotonia, was differentially reinforced for arm and leg movements, i.e. the latter behaviour was reinforced with the sound of her mother's tape-recorded voice while there was no contingency for the former action. In a case of this sort, baselines would be taken on *both* actions, i.e. at (1) in our flow diagram in Figure 3.1 and we would continue recording the nonreinforced behaviour throughout the whole procedure. At (11), of course, it would be possible to return to (1) and begin to reinforce the nontarget behaviour as well. Such an approach is known as a multiple baseline design and ensures that we establish that it is our specific teaching intervention that is producing the observed changes.

Differential reinforcement was also employed with Sian who had suffered postnatal cerebral anoxia and was also spastic quadriplegic with seizures occurring. Here kicking and then head raising were reinforced using a vibratory pad. The last behaviour was particularly relevant to her development as she typically sat with her head on her chest in a flexed position. The developmental advantage of being able to maintain head posture for the development of visual schemes is clear. A physical remedial effect of this sort is also illustrated in the treatment of Mary whose condition was thalamicastrocytoma with mild spasticity. She was first taught to move her right arm to produce music. When the contingency was made available for left arm movement, there was a dramatic change in use of this limb. Brinker and Lewis write:

One effect of Mary's inoperable brain tumour has been general motor impairment which seems more severe on the left side of her body. For example, she will not usually track objects to the left and she shows little movement of her left hand . . . Mary generally held her left hand up to her face with the fist clenched [when] . . . the contingency was reversed from right to left arm . . . the initial effect was that Mary moved her left arm to midline where she moved the left arm by using her right hand . . . she began to move her left arm without the assistance of her right hand. (p. 9)

We can see, then, that in addition to the developmental and motivational advantages of teaching simple Circular Reactions through the use of operant techniques, direct physical advantages can also accrue. However, given the developmental dimension, it is important to consider the direction in which we begin to move to establish more advanced Secondary Circular Reactions that reflect awareness of the different properties of objects in the environment.

In broad development terms the children in Brinker and Lewis's study fell within the Primary Circular Reaction Stage (1–4 months) though the programme had enabled them to develop Secondary Circular Reactions (4–8 months). In Chapter 8 of Volume 1, we described how Glenn and Cunningham (1984), working with similar children, increased the complexity of the contingency analysis task by presenting two stimuli — coloured boxes — only one of which was associated with a potentially reinforcing event, in this case a language-related sound. In the Secondary Circular Reaction period these authors did find that by making the two boxes visually very different, i.e. contrasting their colour and pattern, selective responding could be learnt. It was really at the general developmental level corresponding to the start of Stage IV, Co-ordination of Circular Schemes (8–12 months), that discriminated responding began to emerge. Glenn and Cunningham make the important observation that additional impairments of themselves do not prevent such learning, the critical factor being development at the Stage IV level. From a teaching point of view the study demonstrates the importance of careful structuring of the learning situation and task material. In the case of visually and/or auditorially impaired people comparable variation in the texture could offer the possibility of the pupil picking up on relevant differences. The implications of these authors' findings for classroom practice are described in a further article — 'Special Care — But Active Learning' (Glenn and Cunningham 1985).

In Stage II it is the co-ordination of individual actions and their use in producing an effect on the environment that constitute the main developments. Stephens (1977) offers several practical suggestions to effect these changes:

(i)   The co-ordination of visual tracking of an object with reach and touch. This would be encouraged by directing the child's hand to an object the child was tracking. At this stage touch rather than grasping is all that need be expected.

(ii)   Co-ordination of fixation of an object and touch, e.g. hold aluminium foil in front of the child, then when the foil is fixated guiding the child's hand to it and closing it round the foil then waving the hand with the foil in front of his or her eyes. Fieber suggests extension of this activity with a suitable object being grasped and brought to the child's mouth.

(iii)   Co-ordination of sound and vision by eliciting head turning and visual fixation to two objects waved alternatively on either side of the child.

Fieber emphasises how such co-ordination may present special problems in the motor-impaired child:

> Strong tonic reflex posturing or severe oculomotor problems may interfere with tracking in wide arcs or turning eyes or head to sounds. Due to exaggerated neck extension and abnormal quality of the assymetric tonic neck reflex, the handicapped child's hand may never intersect with his gaze, whereas in the normal child this pattern allows or facilitates hand-watching. Even in the side-lying positioning, neck extension and upward eye deviation combined with extended arms may prevent hand watching. (p. 50)

Similarly, in visually impaired children hand watching may be so close to the eyes that localisation in space does not occur.

While some of the approaches described above involve intensive, one-to-one teaching, others consist of situations in which the person's interaction with equipment, once set up, does not require direct supervision. The flexibility that can be achieved using microtechnology is apparent, but the development of such self-contained systems to enhance early sensorimotor development can be undertaken with more traditional materials.

That people who are profoundly retarded and multiply impaired often do not engage with the world around them will be a familar observation to all those working with this group. Landesman-Dwyer and Sackett (1978) studying 16 such individuals observed that they only spend 5 per cent of their time actively in contact with their environment and only 10 per cent showing overt movement, figures appreciably lower than for nonhandicapped infants and children or individuals who are severely retarded but ambulant. Jones, Favell, Lattimore and Risley (1984) point out that active engagements with objects in the environment is a pre-condition to several aspects of development, citing, among others, Piaget with respect to perceptual and sensorimotor development.

Jones and his colleagues' concern is with devising optimal situations

Figure 3.2: Toy holders: (a) holders with wheelchair table top. Consists of metal rod which is attached to underside of table top. Toys may be positioned at any point along the horizontal frame to encourage midline or lateral arm and head movement. Plexiglas panel prevents toys from moving out of reach when client attempts to grasp, and does not create a visual barrier. Toys may also be fastened to the plexiglas panel: (b) Toyholder attached to the adaptive wheelchair. Holder allows positioning of toys to encourage bilateral midline play, for client with more severe physical limitations.

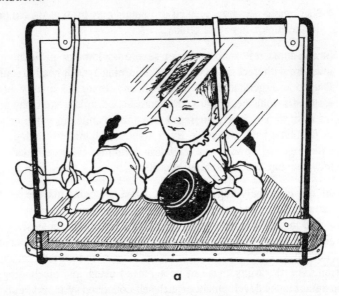

a

in which active engagement is encouraged. They point out that the starting point for creating such situations is the individual's response to the characteristics of the materials employed. They summarise previous unpublished work by Jones (1980) as follows:

> . . . preferences among these clients tend to be idiosyncratic. We have also noted that the density with which toys are available (i.e. providing two or three toys instead of one) can increase levels of independent play. This research has also shown that the method of toy presentation can affect levels of engagement and can also be used to increase or decrease specific behaviours (e.g. increased midline play, reduced mouthing of toys. (Jones *et al.* 1984, pp. 316–17).

On the basis of this work, Jones developed a variety of toy holders to

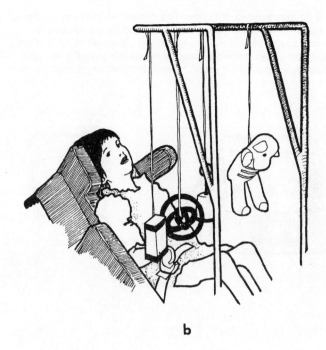

b

Source: Reprinted with permission from *Analysis and Intervention in Developmental Disabilities, 4,* Jones, M.L., Favell, J.E., Lattimore, J. and Risley, T.R. 'Improving Independent Engagement of Nonambulatory Multihandicapped Persons through the Systematic Analysis of Leisure Materials', 1984, Pergamon Press.

be attached to the wheelchair in order to ensure continual availability of objects. These are illustrated in Figures 3.2 and 3.3.

Clearly the actual physical positioning of people in relation to such equipment will be critical and the reader is referred to Fieber's (1977) suggestions below.

The value of these devices for individual clients has been evaluated by Jones *et al.* (1984) with 13 individuals who were profoundly retarded and multiply impaired between CA 8 and 27 years, with an average developmental age of 4.1 months. Three behaviours were observed in the two conditions, i.e. with the toy holder removed and with it present:

(i)   Availability of material — i.e. the engagement material is at least within arm's length.

Figure 3.3: Three-sided Plexiglas Toy Holder with Plywood Base, Attached to Wheelchair Table Top. This apparatus is used in conducting toy evaluations. Toys may be attached to any of the removable plexiglas panels to evaluate positioning of toys, or to all three panels for maximum density and availability of toys.

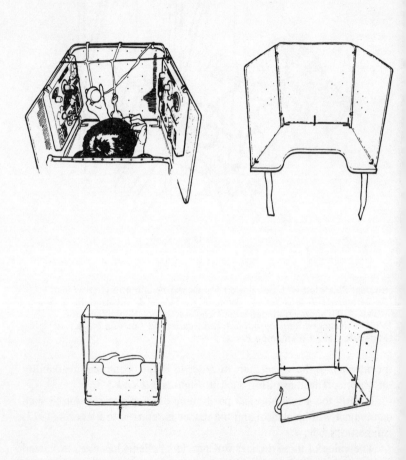

Source: Reprinted with permission from *Analysis and Intervention in Developmental Disabilities, 4,* Jones, M.L., Favell, J.E., Lattimore, J. and Risley, T.R., 'Improving Independent Engagement of Nonambulatory Multihandicapped Persons through Systematic Analysis of Leisure Materials', 1984, Pergamon Press.

(ii)   Engagement with material — touching the object with the palmar side of the hand and moving the object.

(iii)   Engagement by staff — i.e. any form of contact by a staff member.

The actual toys were selected on an individual basis with respect to the factors influencing preference described above, i.e. physical characteristics, number, etc. Most of the material eventually employed was commercially available infant play material appropriate to the individual's developmental age. For example, for one person the material consisted of a jingle bells clutch toy, plastic keys on a ring and an infant chiming rattle.

Introduction of this material led to availability of material 100 per cent of the time in contrast to material availability in the region of 30 per cent prior to its introduction. Following the study proper, Jones *et al.* determined whether staff continued to provide clients with toy holders when not briefed to do so directly. This was found to be the case. For 11 of the 13 clients, the introduction of the toy holders led to an average increase of 41 per cent in engagement, ranging in individuals from 10 to 94 per cent. For five clients, all engagement during the study was observed when the toy holder was present, while for five more, 75 per cent of engagement was during that time. These increases were maintained at follow up. Engagement by staff was not adversely affected by introduction of the toy holders.

What this study does not attempt to demonstrate, and the authors acknowledge the desirability of pursuing the question, is whether actual developmental gains occurred. Did, for example, Primary Circular Reactions give way to Secondary Circular Reactions? Were the forms of grasp refined in any way, and so on? Clearly such changes would have implications for altering the nature of the material provided. Answers to such questions could readily be addressed through observation of the engagement activity itself and independent assessments on developmental scales such as those of Uzgiris and Hunt.

Much of what we have described above will have brought the person to at least the end of Sensorimotor Stage III in a number of the developmental domains. In the following discussion of the various domains we will make it clear where this is the case. In other instances special attention may have to be given to additional Stage I–III behaviours that are not automatically covered in the direct programming of Circular Reactions. In what follows the capital Roman numeral coincides with the equivalent Uzgiris-Hunt and Dunst Scale.

I Visual Pursuit and Permanence of Objects

Here the sighted person will have achieved fixation and tracking of objects, and will visually search for an object that has vanished. The visually impaired person will have developed auditory or tactile equivalents to these behaviours, maintaining contact with the world through hearing and touch. The one behaviour in Stage III that will not have been achieved will be searching for an object that is partially hidden. Here a unitary object in which the person shows interest is partly covered by a piece of material, e.g. a scarf, and is obtained by being pulled from beneath the scarf or removing the scarf and retrieving the object. (Uzgiris Hunt Scale I, critical action code 3c, Dunst Scale step 3.)

The development of programmes to teach object permanence have generally reflected the careful description of steps in the Uzgiris-Hunt Scale. It is important, however, to emphasise that this scale offers a valuable starting point rather than a rigid prescription as to how programming should proceed. There are several reasons for this, reasons that are equally applicable to the other domains we discuss below. First, the various tasks are almost entirely dependent on vision and on manual reaching and grasping. Clearly for many people who are profoundly retarded and multiply impaired, alternative modalities and means of indicating where the object is will be required. Thus, responses to spatial and tactile cues supplemented by audition will have to be worked into the programme as may eye or head pointing in place of reach and grasp. As Fieber (1977) suggests, even in the sighted child difficulties in maintaining eye contact will create problems in the various displacement tasks. Secondly, as she also shows, positioning will be critical:

> The child's chair adaptations need to provide conditions which provide for head stability and centering without any tilt backward of head on body. Because many children's oculomotor control will be more efficient in a centered forward gaze, raising the height of the task presentation will also be helpful. This will also eliminate the dropping forward of the head that may occur with effort to look down at the tray, and the child will maintain better head control. (p. 51)

She goes on to emphasise the co-operation between teacher and physiotherapist in devising tasks that permit 'cognitive' behaviour but also allow the child to use and develop motor abilities. Thirdly, the Uzgiris-Hunt tasks have typically been developed in the context of infants with motivation to explore and interact with the material. Even with such children they allow for flexiblity in testing to ensure that individual differences are taken into account. How much more important, then, is the tailoring of material and consequences to the person who is profoundly retarded and multiply impaired? All that has already been said about establishing effective reinforcers is here applicable. Wherever possible, we will want to ensure that reinforcement is inherent in the task. For example, searching for an object that the person wants in order to produce a sound, such as a bell, is preferable to edible reinforcement in this task. However, the latter should not be rejected out of hand if it proves the most effective way of getting the person into performance on the task.

The starting point in teaching object permanence with people who have attained the necessary prerequisites will be the late Stage III behaviour of reaching for a partially hidden object. Brassel and Dunst (1976), working with low functioning (almost certainly profoundly retarded) people on this task, illustrate how different levels of programming detail can be applied on the initial task (and, of course, on subsequent steps). They contrast 'gross' and 'successive approximation' programming. Here a bright, favoured object, such as doll or plastic object, is to be partially hidden under a scarf. Gross programming involves:

(i)   Holding toy in front of child
(ii)   If it is reached for, then it is placed within easy reach
(iii)   Toy is then covered with cloth so only a part is revealed
(iv)   Child's response is observed and if child accidently recovers toy the sequence is started again

In contrast, successive approximation programming, while beginning with (i) and (ii) above, involves a finer task analysis:

(iii)   The toy is covered approximately 20 per cent so that the cloth is a barrier between child and object
(iv)   If the child gains the object then access to it is allowed for 10 seconds
(v)   This is repeated with approximately 40, 60 and 80 per cent of the toy covered
(vi)   If the child does not uncover the toy on a given trial, then the teacher returns to the previous level of success and introduces even smaller steps.

In their own study, Brassel and Dunst did not find that such fine programming produced any greater improvement than grosser steps. However, in a nonexperimental situation choice of step size will be determined on the basis of the person's performance and points of special difficulty will require increasingly fine analysis until progress is made.

Brassel and Dunst's total programme is available from them, while Kahn (1982) has also provided details of teaching operations that take the pupil through the sensorimotor period in this domain. He also covers partial hiding of an object and moves on to a retrieval of a completely hidden object which should, of course, represent the end stage of a decreasing amount of the toy being visible. With success here, a Level IV behaviour, the programme moves on to hiding on object under one of two screens with the person seeing the object hidden — i.e. visible displacement. Here Stage V is attained and within this stage the teacher can proceed to hiding under three screens. In Stage VI we move to increasingly complex placements in which the person does not actually see the object being placed beneath or behind a given screen. Kahn describes a variety of shaping procedures and successive approximations aimed at taking the pupil to the end of the sensorimotor domain in this area.

Important though this curriculum area is, and possible though it is to teach towards these objectives (see Brassel and Dunst, 1976, 1978; Henry, 1977; Kahn, 1977, 1978, 1982), the issue of maintenance and generalisation is critical. Brassel and Dunst (1976) after effecting changes in a relatively short period show that gains are not maintained after 60 days. For this to occur, then, the pupil must have object-permanence-like experiences on a daily basis. This implies that the teacher must go beyond the highly specific and somewhat artificial teaching situations that ultimately owe their origins to Uzgiris and Hunt's development of Piaget's observations, to either naturally occurring situations or games involving object permanence. The value of such training for object permanence in itself and the development of language resides in its contribution to the pupil's ability to represent absent objects and this development in cognition must be applied beyond the formal teaching situation.

II The Development of Means for Obtaining Desired Objects

All our previous cautionary observations on adapting tasks to the nature of the impairment, positioning and motivation, as well as the need for maintenance and generalisation, apply equally in this domain as in the area of object permanence. With regard to our earlier discussion, the development of Secondary Circular Reactions and visually directed reaching (or an alternative) will have taken the pupil through Sensorimotor Stages I–III. The actions that reflect the progression through Stages IV–VI can be most easily indicated from Dunst's (1980) own summary: Stage IV actions including removing an object to get another desired object; pulling a support such as a piece of cloth on which a desired object has been placed; using some form of locomotion to get an object; Stage V includes not pulling a 'support' when the object is held above it; not pulling either of two 'supports' when the object is between them; pulling a string along a horizontal surface to gain an object; pulling the correct one of two strings to get a desired object; using a string vertically to get an object from the floor; using a stick to obtain a desired object; opening and removing the contents of a matchbox; finding a way of placing a necklace in a matchbox; avoiding stacking a ring that lacks the appropriate hole after trying to do so; Stage VI includes showing foresight in placing a chain in a matchbox; showing foresight by not trying to place a solid ring; using a stick to push a toy out of a transparent tube; and doing the same when the tube is opaque.

It may well be the emphasis on the relation between early language development and the development of the object concept that has led to such an emphasis on teaching object permanence to people with retardation. As we have seen in Chapter 3 of Volume 1, however, the involvement of means-end behaviours also has its advocates. For this reason, Kahn (1982) has included training on means-end behaviour in his programming to teach the cognitive prerequisites of language. Again, the starting point for his programming is encouraging Secondary Circular Reactions and grasping. From there he moves to the Stage IV behaviour of dropping one or both objects in the hands in order to grasp a third. This is achieved through verbal and physical prompting of release and grasping with gradual fading of the prompts. Gaining an object that is on a support is taught through demonstration and prompting again with fading of the prompt. In the next stage a desired object is gradually moved out of reach with prompting to retrieve it at increasing distances. Next, the object is held above the support with the aim of teaching the child to stop pulling the support and reach directly for the object. He recommends that the person be allowed to go on pulling the support for some time so that accommodation can occur. The distance between object and support can be increased to ensure attention to the two objects, then reduced. In subsequent steps prompting and demonstration are employed to teach the child to retrieve an object with a piece of string, both horizontally and vertically. Similar techniques are used to teach retrieval of an object with a stick. The pupil is taught to place a necklace in a container by rolling it up in one hand and steadying the container with the other. If this fails, use of a shorter necklace is advocated with this being progressively increased to the original length. Finally, the stacking task is introduced. Again, Kahn advocates allowing plenty of opportunity for the pupil to learn that the ring without a hole cannot be stacked along with the others. If this is not learned spontaneously, then the holeless ring should be cued to be optimally different from the other rings. For example, while the rings with holes might all be the same colour and shape, the holeless ring should differ on both dimensions. Gradually the differences would be faded until it only differed in the one critical respect, i.e. absence of a hole.

III Development of Gestural Imitation

Though the role of imitation in the acquisition of language varies from child to child, the value of learning new actions through imitation is central in a variety of curricular areas. Certainly, as a formal teaching technique, the use of general imitation plays an important part in most behavioural and co-activation teaching courses. The development of gestural imitation is premised on the fact that the child already emits some gestures spontaneously in a variety of situations. Thus, at Sensorimotor Level II, the pupil will, in Dunst's terms: 'Perform consistent acts in response to familiar, simple gestures (examples: patting table, squeezing a toy, shaking a rattle, banging a table with a spoon)' and will 'Perform consistent acts in response to complex gestures composed of familiar schemes (examples: crumples paper, slides beads, pat-a-cake, hitting blocks together, opening and closing a slinky)'. We will return to actions of these sorts in our discussion of Scale VI object schemes. Here we are concerned with the origins of imitation in Stage III of the sensorimotor period. In Stage III simple, familiar gestures will be imitated with some attempt to imitate complex schemes made up of simple schemes. In Stage IV, complex actions made up of simple schemes and unfamiliar gestures that are visible to the pupil will be imitated. In Stage V an attempt will be made to imitate familiar invisible gestures such as tapping the top of own head or putting out the tongue. Both actions with and without objects will progressively approximate to correct imitations during this stage until two or three invisible actions with and without objects are successfully imitated. At Stage VI the pupil will imitate three invisible gestures without objects.

In several ways this developmental sequence parallels a logical task analysis of the steps to teaching gestural imitation. The movement is from simple to complex, from visible to invisible, and with and without an object. With respect to object use, development will proceed in parallel with object use slightly preceding gestures without an object.

While imitation of movements already made by the person by his or her teacher will represent the earliest type of imitation, the value of imitation training is in the development of more complex and generalised imitation skills. A study by Baer, Peterson and Sherman (1967) illustrates the main features of imitation training. This study was carried out with children, three profoundly and two severely retarded, of 9–12 years of age. None exhibited any imitative behaviour. The model to be imitated was preceded by 'Do this' and a correct imitation was reinforced with food preceded by 'Good'. For the first child the first response was raising the left arm. Initially the teacher prompted this response, i.e. put the child through the movement and then reinforced this prompted response. This prompt was faded by withdrawing the guidance at earlier and earlier points in the movement. In this procedure a time limit was imposed in which the imitation response had to be produced. The complexity of the model was increased throughout training.

Using this technique, separate movements can be chained, i.e. developed as a sequence. In addition, as we shall see, vocal and motor movements can be linked. With the above child, the vocalisation 'Ah!' was linked into the learned motor chain. With another child a progression from blowing out a match to uttering the plosive 'p' was taught.

Within this training procedure an assessment can also be made of whether generalised imitation has developed, i.e. having learnt to imitate certain movements through training, novel models are imitated the first time they are presented. Testing is undertaken by inserting these novel models into the training sequence and not reinforcing such 'probes' even if they are correctly imitated.

Many studies have demonstrated generalised imitation which will also be observed in the natural development of young children. However, there are limits to such generalisation which appears to be restricted to other models coming from the same general class. For example, Garcia, Baer and Firestone (1971) taught imitation of three classes, small motor actions (touch knee, clap hands), large motor (twirl around, touch distant chair) and vocalisations. Generalisation was found to occur *within* any given class (e.g. touch knee to clap hands) but not *between* classes (e.g. not from clap hands to twirl around). (For a fuller technical account of imitation training, see Hogg 1975, pp. 178–81.)

The importance of imitative behaviour in sensorimotor development has already been discussed in Chapter 3 of Volume 1, and training of imitation with individuals who are profoundly retarded will have its place within the curriculum for this stage of development. It will also be obvious, however, that the techniques described above will have application well beyond this stage in a variety of curricular areas discussed in subsequent chapters.

Aspects of the imitation training procedure can also be identified in specialised training procedures that have been developed to teach deaf-blind people and will be discussed later.

IV Operational Causality

The development of means-end behaviour, described earlier, and the development of operational causality, both have their origins in the development of early contingency awareness. Indeed, the first two items on Scale IV (The Development of Operational Causality) relate to the appearance of hand watching and repetition of actions producing an interesting spectacle are also the opening items of Scale II (The Development of Means for Obtaining Desired Environmental Events). However, the scales diverge in that Scale II concerns itself essentially with manipulation of the physical world, e.g. anticipation of the requirement in manipulating physical material, while Scale IV begins to assess what are essentially pragmatic communicative behaviours (see Volume 1, Chapter 3). For example, Scale IV, item 5 is 'passed' if, during demonstration of a spectacle, the child touches an adult and waits during pauses in the spectacle while item 6 can be passed with this behaviour or by the child handing the object back to the adult. The concluding items do, however, return to object manipulation in that attempts to activate a mechanical toy both before and after a demonstration constitute passes.

With respect to teaching, therefore, all that has been written earlier about the development of means-end behaviour in its early, contingency awareness phase, is applicable to the teaching of operational causality. With the somewhat later social context, we are in reality in the early stages of teaching for communication, a clear indication of the intimate relation between early cognition and the development of communication. With respect to this link in the operational causality situation, several general points must be made. First, operational causality with respect to both the activation of spectacles and imperative gestures by the person demands both a motivating spectacle and a sensitive interacting adult. With respect to the spectacle, similar considerations as operate in selection of the reinforcer must be taken into account. The chosen toys or events will probably have been selected from a wide range and the teacher will have closely observed the reactions of pleasure or interest on the pupil's part. Second, sensory impairments will have had to be considered and the event may well be dependent upon one salient form of stimulation, whether auditory, visual or vibratory. Third, it may not initially be possible rigidly to specify what social gesture is to be taken as an indication that the child has developed a pragmatic communication. Of this Fieber (1977) writes:

> It is important not to be arbitrary at this point about either the eliciting situation or the 'procedure' the child chooses. At this level he/she may use different ones for different situations. Observation for any little action on the part of the child can be shaped towards a more systematic signal if one sees the signs of the child continuing to think about the event when it is paused. (p. 55)

With respect to choice of some of the events or toys the later stages of this scale must be borne in mind. The items of the scale are concerned with manipulation of toys by the person to produce an effect. It is therefore important that initial selection of the event takes some account of the present motor competence and limitations of the person. Severe impairment of hand function might preclude a toy or other age-appropriate object having a fine motor component such as turning a small key. However, it is also to be assumed that programmes encouraging motor development will also be in operation and it may be that the operational causality situation can be progressively refined in its demands as motor and physical progress are made.

In the last part of her observation, Fieber refers to the shaping of more systematic gestures or signals that will enable the person to communicate in a way that is standard in that situation. Programmes of this sort may lead into language programmes whether vocal or non-vocal and will be dealt with in the following chapter.

While we are advocating the development of carefully constructed situations in which gestural-vocal causal behaviour can be encouraged, there will be more occasions within the person's day in which the teacher will have the opportunity to respond to signals from the person who is profoundly retarded or by delaying his or her response to give the chance for a communicative response to be emitted (see Chapter 4 for a full discussion of this issue). Once again, the integration of formal teaching aims into the wider framework of the person's life is essential if we are to go beyond a narrowly conceived behavioural curriculum.

V Spatial Development

In Chapter 3 of Volume 1, we described Piaget and Inhelder's (1956) account of spatial development arising from the infant's active interaction with objects in the environment and the importance of movement for the development of perception (Held 1956). We also noted that Piaget's position has been challenged by the view that much information about spatial aspects of the world is given in perception rather than through experience. These positions clearly have implications for our approach to intervention. If the latter is correct, then basic neurological damage to the person who is profoundly retarded and multiply impaired will preclude or severely limit spatial development through intervention.

Though psychologists have yet to resolve this question, we would suggest that adopting the view that spatial understanding *is* constructed through activity has two useful advantages. First, it places the onus on the teacher to concentrate on this important area of development as a curriculum area in its own right. Second, it encourages us to devise clearly thought-out situations in which the child is given the opportunity to act selectively upon different locations in his or her environment, thus utilising whatever perceptual information is available to enhance spatial development.

Though concentrating on spatial development as a curriculum area is of value, it is apparent that in using Uzgiris and Hunt's Scales as a pointer to a curriculum we are already encouraging spatial development in considering several of the other scales. Any item concerned with visual scanning or selective looking reflects the person's ability to respond to different spatial locations. Thus, much of Scale 1 deals with locating objects in space, not only in the early items concerned with visual tracking, but also in later ones in which the person searches for an object beneath various screens. In Chapter 3 of Volume 1, in fact, we pointed out that much of the discussion of spatial development in Stage IV was centred on the child's ability to locate on object beneath one of two screens under varying conditions. Indeed, it could be argued that there is some spatial element in all sensorimotor behaviour even from the earliest behaviours.

While these early developments, e.g. visual tracking, have received attention in discussions of curriculum for people who are multiply handicapped, we find far fewer specific discussions from Stage IV onwards than we do, for example, on development of the object concept. In a sense, the involvement of spatial factors in all other areas tends to lead us to consider that this area is taken care of in passing.

It is worth considering, however, how we can deal more explicitly with the person's relation to the spatial world directly. The experimental literature suggests two important aspects of the teaching situation that can be structured that may enhance the person's understanding of his or her position in space and its relation *to* objects and *between* objects. Experimental studies can be taken as a cue in this respect. Bower (1979) illustrates (Figure 3.4) a simple situation applicable to Stage IV children in which the child's concept of space is based on his or her *own* position in relation to objects (i.e. egocentric spatial behaviour). This is demonstrated by moving the child through differing degrees in relation to objects or moving the objects themselves. In the first picture we see the child seated before three cups, A, B, and C with the object beneath B, in front of the child. When (Picture 2) the child is moved round the table, B, instead of being straight ahead, is to the right. Here reaching for A would indicate spatial egocentrism because the child is reaching on the basis of the object's relation to his or her own position, not to other objects.

A situation of this sort can readily be devised with educational objectives in mind and it is not essential that a hidden object is employed — three distinct objects, reaching for one of which is reinforced, can be employed. Programme objectives can be set which involve the person in reaching for the selected object regardless of the relative positions of the three objects to his or her own position. A shaping procedure is applicable with the person being gradually moved round the table. Similarly, the situation indicated in Picture 3 can also be employed with the child remaining static and the table rotated. According to the work of Butterworth, Jarrett and Hicks (1982) who used a similar situation to that illustrated but with only two objects, it is possible for Stage IV infants to utilise information on the colour of the object and the colour of the surface on which it rests to make the correct choice. In Bower's figure, therefore, we can divide the surface of the table into three contrasting segments in order to provide more information on the correct spatial location.

In the above situation our eventual target behaviours would be 'Person selects correct item regardless of own position or relative positions of objects'. Where the person is mobile, permitting or guiding self-produced movement would be appropriate. Where, however, the person is motorically impaired, less demanding manipulations may be employed. Glenn and Cunningham (1984) advocate use of their PLAYTEST device. Here touch-sensitive boxes at different locations would be employed in a way comparable to the apparatus described by Bower and illustrated in Figure 3.4. A touch, rather than lifting an object, would be the required response and auditory reinforcement or some alternative suitable reinforcer could be the outcome. Where upper limb control is lacking, headpointing or direction of gaze would be alternative responses.

Figure 3.4: After an Object is Placed in the Centre Cup, the Baby is Moved Around the Table or the Table is Turned Around. Either form of movement results in a change of the relative position of the object from centre to right. The baby, however, will still search under the centre cup, demonstrating the egocentrism of his notions of space.

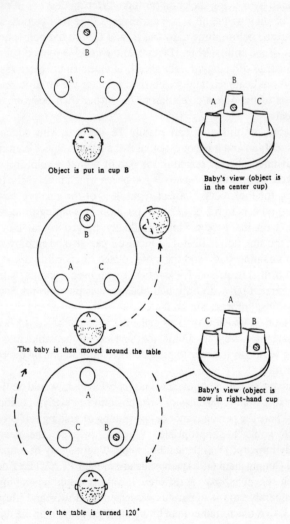

Object is put in cup B

Baby's view (object is in the center cup)

The baby is then moved around the table

Baby's view (object is now in right-hand cup

or the table is turned 120°

Source: Redrawn from Bower, T.G.R. (1979) *Human Development*, W.H. Freeman, San Francisco

Conferring mobility on immobile people is achieved in the above example by moving the pupil round the table. In Chapter 9 of Volume 1 we described Lovett's (1986) use of a modified go-cart, movement of which could be initiated by children who were profoundly retarded and multiply impaired by a simple action (arm or leg movement) breaking a beam. Lovett demonstrated that such a movement was reinforcing to the children who were only at a 2 or 3 month developmental level and were physically impaired. An additional consequence of the child's action was transportation round the room for 10 seconds on each occasion. For those who were not visually impaired, this would lead to changing perceptions of the area through which they travelled, linked, it must be assumed to some changes in proprioceptive and vestibular sensations. For the visually impaired, these last sensations would also be experienced. Though no direct assessment of changes in the child's spatial understanding was attempted by Lovett, his procedure clearly has potential for enhancing this aspect of cognition in a context that does not require constant intervention by a teacher, a further example of the power of microtechnology in enhancing development in this group of people.

In the above discussion we have emphasised the relation between movement and the understanding of spatial relations. Much of Scale V on The Construction of Objects in Space involves the combination of objects — particularly in Dunst's revision. At Stage IV he lists 'Uses hammer-stick to play xylophone', 'Bangs spoon on inverted cup', 'Dumps contents out of a narrow-necked container'; at Stage V: 'Places objects into a cup — dumps out contents', 'Builds tower of two cubes', 'Places rings on stacking stick' and 'Allows object to move down an incline'. Again, we find that teaching objectives often associated with other curricular areas, in this case fine motor or construction items, are seen to have a very specific spatial component. Whether we wish to place items of this kind in the context of this or another curricular area is unimportant. The main concern must be to ensure that the person has experience of relations between objects in space and is given every opportunity to use what means he or she has to manipulate, alter and control these. However, as Fieber (1977) makes clear, our emphasis here is on probing understanding of relations rather than on fine motor ability itself. Motoric assistance is therefore appropriate as in the following illustration: 'For example, in the block stacking item the child may indicate understanding of vertical spatial relationships but be unable to control release'. (Fieber 1977, p. 56).

VI Development of Schemes for Relating to Objects

In its original form this scale was devised to assess typical ways in which infants interact with objects, mainly relatively common toys. Looked at superficially, it is disjointed when compared with, for example, assessment of the object concept or operational causality. Uzgiris and Hunt (1975), however, point to the significance of the various changes that underlie the items in the scale:

At first, objects serve chiefly to elicit various schemes already present within the infant's repertoire of actions. Infants appear to be intent upon exercising these familiar schemes regardless of the characteristics of the eliciting objects. They appear to pay little attention to the characteristics of the objects as such, for the manipulative schemes in the repertoires of very young infants are applied to objects indiscriminately. (p. 122)

Gradually accommodation to the objects takes place. A soft toy is squeezed rather than banged on the table, for example. Emergence of the scheme of examining objects in which an object is looked at while it is manipulated is an important turning point in the object schemes sequence. Here the infant not only shows interest in the features of the object but in appropriate manipulation of it. Schemes now become differentiated taking into account the social significance of the object as well as its physical features. 'Thus, behaviors such as showing objects to a person, including appreciation of their usual function, naming them, and other socially instigated ways of relating to objects come to dominate the actions of the infants in regard to the objects they encounter' (Uzgiris and Hunt 1975 p. 124).

It is important to bear the above description in mind for two reasons. First, simple inspection of the items on the scale does not indicate the true nature of the developmental changes that these items reflect. Second, Piaget has often been criticised for a very abstract account of child development. In this scale the child's understanding of the meaning of objects in themselves and in social settings is assessed and described, i.e. the content of experience is given a central place. As Fieber (1977) puts it: 'The child's spontaneous play with objects reveals the development of the meaning of objects' (p. 58).

Fieber regards this area as one of the most important with respect to low functioning individuals, the expansion of object schemes being a key curricular area. As we have seen, teachers have also taken a special interest in assessing this particular area (e.g. Coupe and Levy 1985). Taking into account the person's interests and abilities, activities are devised that encourage consistent interaction by the child with a range of objects. Demands on accommodation must then be made with novel situations in which adjustment of the scheme (accommodation) is necessary for an effect to be produced. Fieber comments: 'The "same but different" novelty principle will provide general guidance. If the new action is too discrepant with the old, the child will not be able to accommodate his scheme and will lose interest' (p. 59). Variation in material will have the added advantage of sustaining motivation.

A similar principle can be applied as the required schemes move from simple actions to those that are more complex. Thus banging or hitting (Sensorimotor Stage III) will give way to Stage IV complex schemes such as tearing, sliding or swinging. At Stage V social actions with respect to objects will be encouraged. The particular action here will depend upon the object involved. For example, Uzgiris and Hunt (1975 p. 203) list (i) pretending to drink from a cup; (ii) wearing the necklace; (iii) driving the toy car; (iv) building a structure with the blocks; (v) hugging a doll or soft animal; (vi) dressing a doll or putting the shoe on the doll; (vii) sniffing a plastic flower; (viii) making the doll or animal walk (pp. 203–4). There follows 'showing an object to another person' and 'finally naming objects'. While gestural and vocal imitation may play their part in encouraging these later developments in relating to objects, it is obvious that it is exposure to a range of encounters in a social context that will provide the experience for the child to develop in this direction. Clearly any form of deprivation in this respect or isolation from ordinary experiences will be detrimental.

Sensorimotor Teaching and Multiple Sensory Deprivation

In the previous sections we have described possible procedures in teaching sensorimotor development in general with some reference to the adaptation of methods to take account of additional impairments. Consideration must also be given to teaching those who, in McInnes and Treffry's (1982) term, experience *multiple sensory deprivation*. These individuals start basically with visual and auditory impairment which is compounded with sensory deprivation in other modalities arising from lack of vision and sound. In the previous chapter we described briefly the approach advocated by these authors based upon Van Dijk's technique of co-active intervention. McInnes and Treffry's curriculum is based upon traditional areas of functioning, e.g. perception, communication, etc., rather than those divisions suggested by Piagetian theory, and is more akin to a checklist approach in its specification (see Chapter 2). Nevertheless, the aims of their curriculum do embody much that can be derived from the Uzgiris and Hunt Scales in the various developmental domains and we shall illustrate this below.

The starting point for co-active intervention with developmentally young individuals, as described in Chapter 2, is the establishment of a close physical and emotional bond with the person. It is in this context that the teacher encourages and emphasises the integration of sensorimotor activities. The co-activation approach is employed to initiate early sensorimotor actions. With respect to objects, these are placed in the person's hands and co-actively held by the teacher. Varying textures and weights are employed which will encourage accommodation to the varying properties of objects. In parallel to the sensorimotor aspect of this procedure, the co-active therapist is also aiming to develop body awareness. This sequence of interaction follows the path described in Chapter 2. Toleration by the child of adult and object leads to toleration of tactile contact with the object and a growth of interest in the object even if it is not employed for its 'normal' purpose. From here, preference for specific objects over other objects within the same general class emerges. More advanced sensorimotor behaviours will eventually occur involving experimentation and imaginative play. Small objects will be manipulated in a purposive fashion and utilised appropriately. Specific materials play their part in this process and traditional materials such as sand and water are employed.

Much of what appears in McInnes and Treffry's fine motor curriculum (p. 141ff.) also reflects sensorimotor development as described in Piaget and systematised in the Uzgiris and Hunt Scales. For example, their fine motor curriculum begins with the encouragement of reflex grasping (p. 141), a Stage 1 behaviour, and moves on (p. 143) to Primary and Secondary Circular Reactions (p. 143), reflecting Stage II and III behaviours. At these stages too it is possible to select items related to visual tracking and auditory localisation (pp. 167–85 and pp. 198–206 respectively). Co-ordination of schemes is also considered through co-activation at Stage IV with particular emphasis on hand-mouth co-ordination using held and tasted food.

A variety of items in the curriculum deal with the development of object schemes (Uzgiris and Hunt Scale VI). In many instances these are reformulated with respect to tactile rather than visual stimulation. For example, Stage II inspection is dealt with through rotation and touching an object in the hand (7e, p. 145), Stage III exercise of simple schemes by banging (7h, p. 145) and examination, again tactile, through touch (7j, k, p. 145), while dropping appears in items 8a and b (p. 145). This last item and many others are directly comparable to the assessment of spatial development in Scale V of the Uzgiris and Hunt Scales, including those concerned with release of objects and container behaviour.

The approaches developed by Van Dijk and by McInnes and Treffry are applicable to multiply handicapped children across the developmental range, including those whom we would not regard as retarded. Nielsen (1979) has developed a comparable body of techniques aimed more specifically at children who are retarded and blind or partially sighted. She too emphasises the need for the teacher or therapist to have a thorough knowledge of normal developmental processes and patterns. She begins her own interventions early in the sensorimotor period with encouragement of primary schemes through direct contact with the teacher and in a responsive environment. Through playing with the child's own fingers spontaneous activity is encouraged and the teacher must be sensitive to self-initiated activity. Early schemes such as sucking the hands are also encouraged. These self-directed activities are complemented by object-directed activities with an emphasis on grasp, release and retrieval. Sound experiences related to these activities are emphasised in order to bring the child into contact with his or her environment and to develop an experience of space. In developing hand use further, Nielsen advocates making a wide range of objects, two or three dozen, always available to the child in such a way that he or she cannot avoid touching them. Where necessary, physical prompting should be employed.

Nielsen notes that poor head control is often associated with underdeveloped hand use and proposes beginning work where direct contact between child and adult is not involved with the child in the prone position in a responsive setting. Illustratively she suggests:

> Place the infant . . . in a prone position on a platform made of 4mm veneer measuring 1.20 × 1.50 metres. The platform should be raised 2–3 cm above floor level. Then every movement made by the child will not only produce a noise, but the noise will be transmitted by the veneer. By this means the sound quality of the child's activity will be reinforced, and there is a good chance that the child will be able to sense it and be inspired to make further movements. Gradually the child will understand the sounds he hears are sounds that he is creating himself. (p. 11)

By placing an object under the child's head, such as a plastic plate, head movements will naturally produce sound. By rubbing the plate with orange or vanilla, experiences of smell or taste can result from movement.

Participation with an adult in everyday activities accompanied by verbal descriptions is suggested. These activites can embrace shutting doors, switching on lights, turning taps and so on: '. . . in short, all the noise making activities which are being engaged in in the course of the day in an everyday home-life situation.' (p. 17). Nielsen emphasises the need to relate all play activities to participation in everyday care situations such as eating and bathing 'so that a natural relationship is established between play and everyday situations', (p. 26).

It may be seen, therefore, that the basic sensorimotor developments that we have described earlier in this chapter are equally relevant to deaf-blind children in this stage of development. The technique of co-active intervention is a usable approach that is perfectly consistent with the specification of clear objectives and makes special provision for breaking through the isolation that must be experienced by multiply sensorily deprived individuals living, as Van Dijk (1977) suggests, 'in a shell which is their own body'.

In indicating the relations between McInnes and Treffry's curriculum and the organisation suggested by Piagetian domains we are not advocating that their approach should necessarily be reformulated in these terms, only that the co-active technique is shown by them to be highly applicable to the individuals with whom we are concerned in the sensorimotor stage. A similar conclusion may be drawn with respect to early preoperational development, a topic to which we shall shortly turn.

A final word on sensorimotor programming: At the present stage of development in evolving a curriculum at the sensorimotor level for people who are profoundly retarded and multiply impaired, we have found it helpful to organise curricular areas in close concordance with Uzgiris and Hunt's domains of assessment. We have tried to make it clear, however, that there is much interdependence between these domains, that, for example, development of the object concept and spatial development are far from entirely distinct. We have also suggested that with the lowest functioning individuals, our starting point can be with Primary and Secondary Circular Reactions that form the basis of more complex behaviour as it becomes differentiated. Finally, we have emphasised that much of the content of a sensorimotor curriculum can be realised through systematic behavioural programming and where relevant through co-active intervention techniques. As our concluding observation in a previous section urged, however, the need for social interaction in ordinary social contexts ultimately supplied the content of experience that permits more advanced development.

It is, of course, this content that will be represented symbolically at around Sensorimotor Stage VI and will permit both symbolic play and the emergence of language. We will return to the latter in the following chapter but will here move on to the encouragement of play and activities suitable to the preconceptual stage of the preoperational period.

Preoperational Teaching Objectives

We saw in Chapter 7 of Volume 1, that assessment in the preoperational period of children with mental handicap is not as well developed as for sensorimotor domains. Nevertheless, several approaches to such assessment were noted, and become of relevance as the individual nears the end of Sensorimotor Stage VI. In like vein, curricular development in the preoperational period is less adequately developed for individuals who are profoundly retarded and specific studies are few and far between. Stephens (1977) notes that as we move into this period we are going to be increasingly dependent upon more conventional nursery curricula, though clearly additional impairments will require a range of modifications to teaching material.

In what follows we deal briefly with the conditions under which symbolic play can be encouraged and describe one strategy in relation to teaching basic preoperational developments in the areas of classification, number, measurement and space, and seriation. With respect to the former, we will consider suggestions made in the context of a more general consideration of play of mentally handicapped children by Jeffree, McConkey and Hewson (1977). With regard to general cognitive development, we follow Stephens (1977) in suggesting that the work of Lavatelli (1970a and b) provides a well-structured approach to teaching and materials that can be adapted to the needs of the multiply impaired retarded child.

Symbolic Play

Clearly the range of different types of play in which any child can engage or be engaged go beyond symbolic play and occur in a variety of situations that might naturally occur in other areas of the curriculum. Jeffree *et al.* distinguish and discuss exploratory play, energetic play, skilful play, social play, imaginative play and 'puzzle it out play'. Much of the discussion of early exploratory play is concerned with what has here been referred to as Piaget's mastery play in the sensorimotor period and has been considered in this chapter in terms of contingency awareness, the development of the object concept, object schemes and causality. Jeffree *et al.'s* energetic play subsumes a variety of gross motor developments dealt with here and later in Chapter 5, where fine motor skills, Jeffree *et al.'s* 'skilful play', will also be covered. Social play reflects parent- (or teacher-)child interactions and will be considered in the following chapter. It is in their last two sections that these authors focus directly on the preoperational period. 'Puzzle it out' play is concerned with several major preoperational developments including those in the areas of seriation and classification. Imaginative play deals directly with symbolic play activities, many of them directly comparable to the situations employed in Lowe and Costello's (1976) play assessment battery. Jeffree *et al.* make the important point that in all these areas, advances can be encouraged through play-like activities. These can be employed to complement more direct teaching and therapy as opportunities occur, or are created, in naturally occurring interactions. Within the scope of this chapter, however, it is their discussion of symbolic play that is of particular relevance and with which we will deal in more detail.

Jeffree *et al.'s* suggestions regarding symbolic play deal with (i) the pupil as initiator; and (ii) the teacher as scene setter. With respect to the former they emphasise that in its early stages symbolic play may be fleeting, e.g. a cup is put briefly to the mouth. In addition, physical impairment may create difficulty in the very attempt to make the action, resulting in its imperfect realisation. Thus, sensitive observation is called for. With regard to the latter, the teacher should, in advance, create clearly structured situations in which material with the potential for eliciting symbolic play is available. These authors also note, however, that in its early stages it may be necessary to employ imitation teaching in order to encourage symbolic actions. This would begin with actions directed towards the self, e.g. related to eating or drinking, and be followed by, for example, doll play in which basic actions such as kissing or cradling would be modelled. Again the possibility of deferred imitation emphasises the need for sensitive observation following the immediate imitation session. The nature of the material and the complexity of the play is then extended as spontaneous symbolic play is observed.

With respect to the generalisation of these suggestions for encouraging symbolic play in people who are retarded with additional impairments we are thrown back on broad prescriptions that underpin all intervention with this group. For the person with restricted mobility and poor postural control, play settings will have to be created *in situ* and adequate support given. Limitations in vision and hearing will have to be taken into account and co-active techniques of the sort advocated by McInnes and Treffry (1982) for use with deaf-blind children employed. The detailed working out of play settings to encourage the development of symbolic play in people who are profoundly retarded and multiply impaired is a neglected area of the curriculum and one which merits considerable attention in order to provide approaches that complement and extend the basic behavioural techniques with which we are more familiar.

Cognition

The basic nursery materials that reflect and encourage development in the preoperational period are by now familar to all teachers and to most parents. We noted earlier (p. 90) Stephens' (1977) comment on the need to adapt existing teaching resources to the aims of the sensorimotor curriculum. This same state of affairs holds, too, for the preoperational curriculum.

In order to give a clear impression of the content of such a curriculum and the specific teaching concerns involved we will draw upon one such curriculum. This is Lavatelli's and is chosen because (i) its theoretical basis in Piaget's work is clearly stated and is consistent with the development of Piagetian applications in the field of profound retardation described in this book; (ii) both materials and objectives are clearly stated; (iii) it emphasises development of understanding beyond the immediate teaching context in natural settings and thus addresses the issues of generalisation and ecological validity of the teaching; (iv) it suggests complementary language activities in the context of teaching a range of cognitive skills.

Lavatelli (1970a) has outlined a curriculum based on the main domains of development during the preoperational period and has coordinated this with a teacher's guide (Lavatelli, 1970b) and a materials kit for use in the various curricular areas. The value of this three-pronged approach — theory, curricular content and materials — should not be under-emphasised, though as will be clear from our brief descriptions of the materials, these can readily be assembled from a variety of early educational material catalogues or in some cases produced by a teacher or parent.

Lavatelli's approach recommends small group work with three or four children in quiet areas of the classroom. In considering its use with people who are profoundly retarded it is likely that adaptation to the more typical one-to-one situation will be called for. Similarly, length of any session must be tailored to the attention span of the individual. While specific material is recommended for these teaching sessions, an emphasis is placed on generalisation to nonteaching sessions and settings in which everyday tasks demand the same understanding are suggested. The main teaching areas are as follows:

Classification. (i) Identifying properties of objects and matching one-to-one correspondence. Here coloured beads are employed and development is towards multiple classification, i.e. where two criteria have to be employed in order to classify.

(ii) Complementary classes. Here the emphasis is on identifying subclasses and classes, flexibility of grouping, and complementary classes, e.g. where the class of red trucks complements the overall class of trucks. Material here is toy cars, trucks and aeroplanes of varying sizes, and colours, as well as nontransport items.

(iii) Class inclusion. Here classes are combined to make a superordinate class and reversal to compare parts of a class with its whole encouraged. Material consists of toy dogs and cats of varying colours.

(iv) Hindsight and foresight. Here mental operations concerning figuring out what objects have in common and using these as the basis of grouping is the focus. Miniature toys such as eating utensils, plastic animals and a toy tool set are used.

(v) Intersection of classes. Here it is necessary to keep the common property of each of two groups of objects in mind while selecting objects with both characteristics. In this, wooden shapes of varying colours can be employed.

(vi) Combinations and permutations. For example, items that go together, doll's sweater and skirt for example, are presented — two sweaters and two skirts. The child has to discover how many outfits can be made from this number. Girl and boy doll sets and train sets are employed here.

Number, Measurement and Space. (i) Conservation of number. This begins with establishing one-to-one correspondence and upsetting the equivalence by adding or subtracting items and encouraging the person to restore equivalence. Here miniature objects and coins are employed.

(ii) Conservation of number — one-to-one correspondence without physical correspondence. In addition, the concept of a half is taught by dividing equally the material which consists of wooden cubes and of pipe cleaners.

(iii) Conservation of liquid quantity. Liquid is presented in various containers and manipulated between them noting that change in one dimension can be compensated for by change in another. Equivalence is established through reversal of operations, i.e. tipping liquid from A to B and back again. Material here consists of cylinders of various sizes and shapes, a plastic funnel and a shallow dish.

(iv) Conservation of quantity with and without visual correspondence. Here sets of objects are compared in which following demonstration of one-to-one correspondence, the objects are placed in different shaped containers when the objects can be seen and when they cannot. Here marbles are employed in conjunction with plastic containers and bags.

(v) Horizontal and vertical reference points. Achieved through drawing lines on outline pictures of flasks to indicate water level. Tilting from vertical also employed. Material includes transparent screw top flask.

(vi) Conservation of surface area. Taught through use of cardboard 'fields' on which toy cars can be placed. 'Have the children upset the equivalence of the grass area by "parking" a car on one field . . .?' (p. 57). The operation can be reversed to establish equivalence of area; parts of field can be rearranged to achieve conservation.

(vii) Conservation of length and introduction to measurement. Here parts are combined into wholes by putting parts together in different ways to make equal wholes. Identification of a unit as part of a whole is also required. Foam blocks of varying size for tower buildings with equivalent towers built from bases at different heights and rods are employed to establish equivalence of height.

(viii) Spatial transformations. These situations are natural extensions of those described earlier in this chapter on encouraging spatial development in the sensorimotor period. Transformations of position through 180° in relation to a left-hand position of items is employed. The situation suggested is a place setting of knife and fork with the child matching the relative positions (fork right, knife left) to a completed setting on the opposite side of the table.

(ix) Spatial representation. Here a house, tree and garage model is employed. The pupil is shown one of four pictures of what this model looks like when viewed from any given side and has to indicate understanding of the view seen from that side.

Seriation. (i) Seriation of length with insertion of a new unit. Here basic seriation, i.e. ordering of, for example, rods of varying length is taught plus placement of a rod at the appropriate point in an already completed sequence. Though we have referred to a rod, Lavatelli's material actually consists of cut-out flower pots of varying size.

(ii) Seriation of two sets of objects. Here identification of comparable items from within two series is called for, e.g. selection of the largest doll in a series and of the largest umbrella.

(iii) Seriation of length and colour. Here two criteria for ordering are employed, e.g. variation in size *and* brightness. Strips of coloured paper are employed here.

(iv) Multiple seriation. Here, for example, geometric shapes are seriated by size and number of sides.

(v) Transitivity. Here an area puzzle set is employed in which the aim is to recognise that if it takes more units to cover area A than it does Area B then A is a larger area than B.

Throughout this teaching an emphasis is placed on parallel language and Lavatelli suggests the form that this may take. For example, in classification the recognition that the classes of animals is larger than the classes of dogs *and* cats which make it up is complemented by the use of such comparatives as 'more' and 'bigger' and pronouns such as 'all' and 'some'. In the Number, Measurement and Space domain conservation of length and the introduction of measurement elicits the vocabulary for comparing length — 'taller than', 'higher than', 'shorter than', etc., and prepositions such as 'on top' or 'under'. In seriation of length with insertion of a new unit, for example, terms such as 'biggest' and 'smallest' would be employed. With respect to generalisation to everyday situations, Lavatelli suggests a number of relevant contexts. Classification of food items can be recognised at snack time where opportunities of illustrating conservation of liquid also present themselves. Seriation can be emphasised in nursery stories such as *The Three Bears*.

It will already have been noticed that although the continuity with the sensorimotor developments described is maintained in Lavatelli's preoperational curriculum, it takes us well beyond the expectations we have for many of those individuals we regard as profoundly retarded and multiply impaired. Nevertheless, in gearing our teaching of cognition to this continuum we ensure that (i) we know where we hope to be going in terms of long-term aims and (ii) avoid a dangerous implicit assumption regarding the person's limitations. Thus we teach towards these more advanced aims however slow the progress.

With respect to rate of learning beyond the achievement of full sensorimotor development, we will need to make many adaptations to the form of Lavatelli's methods. At the early preoperational stage, for example, the teaching of matching may involve careful programming of both discrimination between objects and subsequent match-to-sample. We will be drawing on the extensive literature on techniques for such teaching and limiting the size of teaching steps just as we did in the case of simple Circular Reactions. Working with adults who were generally in the early stage of preoperational development (Developmental ages 2 to 3 years), Richmond and Bell (1983) showed how careful cueing could be employed to teach size discrimination and the advantage of cueing techniques over trial and error learning.

The observations we made on the effect of traditional impairments following our discussion of symbolic play should also be borne in mind. Adaptation of Lavatelli's standard nursery material will be called for where physical or sensory impairment reduces the person's ability to manipulate it or experience it. Nielsen's approach, described above in relation to the sensorimotor period, is extended to the preoperational period. Here the emphasis is on creating situations in which concepts such as similar and different can be developed and in which classification is encouraged through sorting activities. Parallel use of language to describe what is happening is also employed as in Lavatelli's work. Techniques explicitly aimed at individuals who are blind or partially sighted are suggested. Where older individuals are concerned, attention should be paid to the development of material that is age-appropriate. Here everyday activities for older people need to be considered in relation to the academic side of cognitive teaching.

In both the sensorimotor and the preoperational areas of the curriculum discussed, we have referred to the development of communication and language. It is to this topic as a central concern in the development of people who are profoundly retarded and multiply impaired that we now turn.

References

Baer, D.M., Peterson, R.F. and Sherman, J.A. (1967) 'The Development of Imitation by Reinforcing Behavioral Similarity to a Model', *Journal of the Experimental Analysis of Behavior, 10,* 405–16

Bower, T.G.R. (1979) *Human Development,* W.H. Freeman, San Francisco

Brassel, W.R. and Dunst, C.J. (1976) 'Comparison of Two Procedures for Fostering the Development of the Object Construct', *American Journal of Mental Deficiency, 80,* 523–8

Brassel, W.R. and Dunst, C.J. (1978) 'Fostering the Object Construct: Large-scale Intervention with Handicapped Infants', *American Journal of Mental Deficiency, 87,* 507–10

Brinker, R.P. and Lewis, M. (1982a) 'Contingency Intervention in Infancy' in J. Anderson and J. Cox (eds.), *Curriculum Materials for High Risk and Handicapped Infants,* Technical Assistance and Development System, Chapel Hill. N.C.

Brinker, R.P. and Lewis, M. (1982b) 'Discovering the Competent Infant: A Process Approach to Assessment and Intervention', *Topics in Early Childhood*

Special Education, 2 (2)

Brinker, R.P. and Lewis, M. (1982c) 'Making the World Work with Microcomputers: A Learning Prosthesis for Handicapped Infants', *Exceptional Children, 49*, 163–70

Butterworth, G., Jarrett, N. and Hicks, L. (1982) 'Spatiotemporal Identity in Infancy: Perceptual Competence or Conceptual Deficit', *Developmental Psychology, 18*, 435–49

Coupe, J. and Levy, D. (1985) 'The Object Related Scheme Assessment Procedure: A Cognitive Assessment for Developmentally Young Children who may have Additional Physical or Sensory Handicaps', *Mental Handicap, 13*, 22–4

Dunst, C.J. (1980) *A Clinical and Educational Manual for Use with the Uzgiris and Hunt Scales of Infant Psychological Development*, Pro-Ed, Inc., Austin, Tex.

Fieber, N.M. (1977) 'Sensorimotor Cognitive Assessment and Curriculum for the Multihandicapped Child' in J. Cronin (ed.), *The Severely and Profoundly Handicapped Child*, State Board of Education, Illinois

Fuller, P.R. (1949) 'Operant Conditioning of a Vegatative Human Organism', *American Journal of Mental Deficiency, 62*, 587–90

Garcia, E. Baer, D.M. and Firestone, I. (1971) 'The Development of Generalized Imitation within Topographically Determined Boundaries', *Journal of Applied Behavior Analysis, 4*, 101–12

Glenn, S.M. and Cunningham, C.C. (1984) 'Selective Auditory Preferences and the Use of Automated Equipment by Severely, Profoundly and Multiply Handicapped Children', *Journal of Mental Deficiency Research, 28*, 281–96

Glenn, S.M. and Cunningham, C. (1985) 'Special Care-But Active Learning', *Special Education: Forward Trends, 11*, 33–6

Held, R. (1956) 'Plasticity in Sensory-motor Systems', *Scientific American, 213*, 84–94

Henry, J.C. (1977) 'The Effects of Parent Assessment and Parent Training on Preschool Mentally Retarded Children on Piagetian Tasks of Object Permanence', unpublished dissertation, Temple University, Philadelphia

Hogg, J. (1975) 'The Experimental Analysis of Retarded Behaviour and its Relation to Normal Development' in M.P. Feldman and A. Broadhurst (eds.), *Theoretical and Experimental Bases of the Behaviour Therapies*, Wiley, London and New York

Hogg, J. (1983) 'Sensory and Social Reinforcement of Head-turning in a Profoundly Retarded Multiply Handicapped Child', *British Journal of Clinical Psychology, 22*, 33–40

Jeffree, D.M., McConkey, R. and Hewson, S. (1977) *Let Me Play*, Souvenir Press, London

Jones, M.L. (1980) 'The Analysis of Play Material for the Profoundly Retarded', unpublished master's thesis, University of Kansas, Lawrence, Ks.

Jones, M.L., Favell, J.E., Lattimore, J. and Risley, T.R. (1984) 'Improving Independent Engagement of Nonambulatory Multihandicapped Persons through the Systematic Analysis of Leisure Materials', *Analysis and Intervention in Developmental Disabilities', 4*, 313–32

Kahn, J.V. (1977) 'On Training Generalized Thinking', Paper presented at American Psychological Association, San Francisco

Kahn, J.V. (1978) 'Acceleration of Object Permanence with Severely and Profoundly Retarded Children', *American Association for the Severely/Profoundly Handicapped Review, 3*, 273–80

Kahn, J.V. (1982) Cognitive Training and its Relationship to the Language of Profoundly Retarded Children', Final Report to the Illinois Department of Mental Health and Developmental Disabilities, University of Illinois at Chicago, Chicago, Ill.

Landesman-Dwyer, S. and Sackett, G. (1978) 'Behavior Changes in Non-ambulatory, Mentally Retarded Individuals' in C.E. Myers (ed.), *Quality of Life in Severely and Profoundly Mentally Retarded People: Research Foundations for Improvement,* American Association on Mental Deficiency, Washington, D.C.

Lavatelli, C.S. (1970a) *Early Childhood Curriculum — A Piaget Program,* American Science and Engineering Company, Boston

Lavatelli, C.S. (1970b) *Teacher's Guide to Accompany Early Childhood Curriculum,* American Science and Engineering Company, Boston

Lovett, S. (1986) 'An Experiment to Investigate Discrimination Learning in Multiply Handicapped Children Using an Electromechanical Chair' in P. Sturmey, J. Hogg and A. Crisp (eds.), 'Organising Environments for People with Mental Handicap', submitted for publication

Lowe, M. and Costello, A.J. (1976) *Manual for the Symbolic Play Test Experimental Edition,* NFER-Nelson, Windsor

McInnes, J.M. and Treffry, J.A. (1982) *Deaf-blind Infants and Children: A Developmental Guide,* University of Toronto Press, Toronto/Open University Press, Milton Keynes

Nielsen, L. (1979) *The Comprehending Hand,* Refsnaesskolen, State School for Blind and Partially Sighted Children, Copenhagen

Piaget, J. and Inhelder, B. (1956) *The Child's Conception of Space,* Routledge and Kegan Paul, London

Piper, T.J. and MacKinnon, R.C. (1969) 'Operant Conditioning of a Profoundly Retarded Individual Reinforced via a Stomach Fistula', *American Journal of Mental Deficiency, 73*, 627–30

Remington, R.E. (1975) 'Auditory Reinforcement in Profoundly Retarded Multiply Handicapped Children' in J. Hogg, T. Foxen and R.E. Remington, *Research into the Assessment and Remediation of Behavioural Deficits in Profoundly Retarded Multiply Handicapped Children,* Hester Adrian Research Centre, University of Manchester, Manchester

Remington, R.E., Foxen, T. and Hogg, J. (1977) 'Auditory Reinforcement in Profoundly Retarded Multiply Handicapped Chidren', *American Journal of Mental Deficiency, 82,* 299–304

Richmond, G. and Bell, J. (1983) 'Comparison of Three Methods to Train a Size Discrimination with Profoundly Retarded Students', *American Journal of Mental Deficiency, 87,* 574–6

Stephens, B. (1977) 'A Piagetian Approach to Curriculum Development for the Severely, Profoundly and Multiply Handicapped' in E. Sontag, J. Smith and N. Certo (eds.), *Educational Programming for the Severely and Profoundly Handicapped,* Division of Mental Retardation, Reston, VA.

Uzgiris, I.C. and Hunt, J. McV. (1975) *Assessment in Infancy: Ordinal Scales of Psychological Development,* University of Illinois Press, Urbana

Van Dijk, J. (1977) 'What we Have Learned in 12½ Years: Principles of Deaf-Blind Education' in M.R. Jurgens (ed.), *Confrontation Between the Young Deaf-Blind Child and the Rest of the World*, Swets and Zeitlinger, Lisse

4 DEVELOPING COMMUNICATION

Introduction

Central to any curriculum directed to people with severe learning difficulties will be the aim of facilitating their ability to communicate. As in other areas of development, people with profound retardation will show massive delays in communication, often complicated by additional sensory and physical impairments.

The term 'communication' is employed to cover the many different ways in which one person can convey to others his or her experiences of the world. Conventionally this is done through spoken language, usually accompanied by facial expressions and bodily movements. It is equally possible, however, to communicate without speech, i.e. non-orally. This we often do in our daily lives through gestures, and we have seen in Chapter 5 of Volume 1 how hearing-impaired children will often invent their own private sign-languages. Such non-oral communication systems can, of course, be formalised into manual sign languages and a variety of other systems that permit non-spoken communication.

We will first deal in this chapter with programmes intended to teach or enhance spoken language and prerequisites for such development. Then we will briefly consider the problem of eliminating inappropriate vocalisations. Finally, we will consider what decisions should be taken if progress to spoken language is unacceptably slow. Here the issue of non-oral communication systems is dealt with and the choice of available systems considered.

While research into language teaching for nonverbal people has been carried out with great intensity over the past 20 years, there has been continual revision of ideas as to how it should be undertaken. These revisions have stemmed from two sources. First, careful evaluation of language programmes has pointed to shortcomings in their effectiveness that require alternative approaches to the problem. Second, changing views on the nature of child development in general and language acquisition in particular have suggested new ways of approaching language intervention. Both of these sources of change affect language intervention for all nonverbal groups, including those who are profoundly retarded and multiply impaired. For this reason we will begin the chapter not by describing programmes in their developmental sequence, i.e.

programmes from the least able upwards, but by considering the basic language training paradigm that emerged during the 1960s, and then considering how it has been developed and altered to take account of its demonstrable shortcomings. Against this background we can then consider how the special needs of those with profound retardation and multiple impairments can be met within the revised framework.

Teaching Spoken Language

During the period with which we are concerned, over 200 programmes for language-delayed or -disordered people have been developed. Many of these have been directed to people with retardation and a majority have employed behavioural teaching techniques. In a review of the first ten years of this period Harris (1975) describes the main features of behavioural language programmes and some of the limitations that have emerged to which other research workers have responded. In order to understand the direction later work has taken, we will briefly summarise Harris's main observations.

Harris describes the typical sequence of a behavioural language teaching programme as consisting of four phases: attention; nonverbal imitation; verbal imitation; and functional speech.

Attention figures as the starting point for such programmes since attention to the teacher is regarded as the first prerequisite for language learning. Typically, teaching attending-behaviour is undertaken with the adult facing the learner, sometimes in an individual teaching room and sometimes in the open classroom. A well-established pattern of obtaining eye contact is developed consisting of reinforcement of spontaneous eye contact or prompting attention, then reinforcing the behaviour. Duration of attention can then be extended through appropriate shaping. Harris also noted less formal attempts to establish attention.

When the person is attending to the teacher, behaviour is brought under imitative control. Usually such teaching begins with gross motor imitation, e.g. holding the arms in the air or standing up, in response to the teacher's verbal instruction: 'Do this!' followed by the model to be imitated. As Harris points out, there is little evidence that such a procedure is essential as a requirement for entering a language programme. Evidence does suggest that learning gross motor imitation does not facilitate vocal imitation and the transition is often an extremely difficult one. With respect to verbal imitation, relatively standard procedures have again been developed consisting of: (i) reinforcing all vocalisations; (ii) reinforcing vocalisations that imitate the teacher's model within a preset number of seconds; (iii) reinforcing vocalisations that approximate the teacher's vocalisation; (iv) introducing new sounds to be imitated. This approach can be undertaken in one-to-one settings and with groups, and many reports have attested to its effectiveness as a teaching method. Assistance is given to the learner through prompting and cueing, with eventual fading of prompts and cues as he or she becomes more proficient. Harris notes that despite the many reports of successful teaching of verbal imitation, there are a few that indicate failure. She speculates that many more may not have been published and that it is possible that there are individuals in whom biological damage actually prevents the learning of speech, a point particularly relevant when considering teaching techniques for the group with whom we are concerned here.

In the fourth phase the behavioural teacher moves on to teaching what Harris refers to as functional speech. Typically such training begins with teaching nouns to label specific objects or illustrations of objects. Progressively more complex forms of syntax can be taught and she lists: expressive and receptive plural nouns, receptive prepositions, singular and plural declarative sentences, verb tenses, adjectival inflections, compound sentences, complex sentences, interrogative sentences and so on. In addition, a central concern at this stage relates to generalisation and maintenance of learned behaviour. Do the grammatical forms learnt with specific words and objects generalise to new words and objects? For example, if the child has learnt to say 'Spoon' to a single spoon and 'Spoons' to two spoons, and 'Fork' to a single fork will she say 'Forks' on first being presented with two such implements without having been taught to use this plural form? Similarly, generalisation across individuals and locations is of concern. Does the child employ the learned forms in the presence of a person not involved in the initial teaching and in other locations than, for example, the individual teaching room? Once learning and generalisation have been achieved, are they maintained over time, at least with respect to months if not years?

The above strategy, with some variation, has been incorporated into a range of language teaching programmes, some of extensive detail. All draw explicitly or indirectly on our knowledge of norm sequences of development with their obvious feature that language becomes more complex as children get older. Within this broad tradition of work, for example, Guess, Sailor, Keogh and Baer (1976) have elaborated an extensive language development programme for children with severe handicaps. In the light of their success with programming strategies of the kind described above, they set out to evolve a comprehensive intervention programme for individuals who are nonverbal or seriously speech deficient. Since the formal starting point for their programme assumes that the student has verbal imitation skills, then clearly an assessment showing he or she was deficient in this respect would require some training prior to entry into the main programme. In relation to sensorimotor assessment and programming, this entails bringing the student to Stage V and VI functioning employing techniques summarised above from Harris (1975). In relation to seriously motor-impaired or hearing-impaired people with profound retardation, this strategy would be precluded and alternative approaches to the initiation of communication would have to be considered.

Guess *et al.* (1976) summarise one programmed instruction package devised by Tawney and Hipsher (1972) specifically aimed at low functioning individuals who emit no vocal or motor responses. This was devised for teachers who are relatively inexperienced in the area of teaching communication and employs operant techniques. Sequences of target behaviours are specified as are the required prerequisites for entry to each step and pre and post test assessments to evaluate the success of the teaching. The general sequence of instruction as outlined by Guess *et al.* is as follows:

(1) shape attending behavior in tutorial sessions; (2) shape other skills, such as the touch response, which are prerequisite to further instruction; (3) teach concepts at the motor level through a discrimination learning procedure; (4) establish speech sounds; (5) shape sounds into one word responses; (6) teach 'touch' in conjunction with vocal responses; (7) fade instructions, and teach concepts at the verbal level; (8) expand one-word utterances to two and three words; (9) combine noun and verb phrases; and (10) reinforce spontaneous utterances.

Clearly this sequence overlaps with the programme devised by Guess *et al.* Their programme covers ten content areas which begin with core elements for all students and which are 'Persons and Things' and 'Actions with persons and things'. The programme then branches into preacademic areas (possession, colour, size and relation) and Community living (social skills, help-seeking and conversational speech). This last is designed explicitly to assist those 'who need specific, direct training in language skills facilitating life in their home, or in a community sheltered workshop, half-way house, nursing home, or any other setting where basic social and survival communication skills assume a major importance' (pp. 305–6). Within each content area the sequence of training steps are organised with respect to the symbolisation of events or objects in language, i.e. reference to events and objects, control of the environment through productive language ('I want . . .') and receptive language ('yes' in response to a query), self-extended control, i.e. asking for further information in the way described in Volume 1, Chapter 3, integration entailing the chaining of previously learned skills centred on some activity, and receptive language as an essential complement to productive language which the programme emphasises.

The Guess *et al.* programme within this framework specifies training goals, stimulus material, instructions to the trainer and also detailed procedures for teaching generalisation. For the purpose of this chapter it is not necessary to elaborate further on either Tawney and Hipsher's or Guess *et al.'s* programmes or the specific aspects of behavioural techniques employed in such programmes. We have spent a little time describing this general framework in order to be able to consider its relevance to individuals with profound retardation and multiple impairments and in order to demonstrate how shortcomings in the approach arising from it have been dealt with by teachers and research workers in this field.

Much of the published work employing the behavioural approach to language teaching has been directed to individuals falling within the severe to profound range of retardation. Its downward extension has been limited by two obvious factors to which we have already referred. First, the developmental cognitive factors that are prerequisites for entry into communication skills and which evolve in the preoperational stage of development are often lacking in the population with which we are concerned. Second, motor and sensory impairments preclude the 'natural' progression through imitation training to more complex forms of communication. With respect to the first limitation, the implication is that we specifically teach the cognitive prerequisites and we have seen in the previous chapter how we can devise programmes that advance individuals whose sensorimotor performance was insufficiently high to enter a conventional language programme. Later in this chapter we will emphasise the continuity of sensorimotor and language programmes. With respect to the second, the degree of impairment will determine whether we can proceed with language programmes of the sort described above. Not all forms of physical impairment or degrees of visual or auditory impairment preclude entry into such a programme. In relation to these two classes of imitation, then, there will be individuals with profound retardation and multiple impairments for whom we will have to devise quite distinct approaches to communication intervention. For others, however, we will be able to engage in more formal language teaching. In this last case, we wish to consider not only language packages of the sort described, but also developments to them that have come into being through failures in their implementation. At this point, however, we will consider some of the few published studies that consider individuals with profound retardation within the above behavioural framework. In none of these were the students seriously impaired physically or sensorily. The studies chosen cover the use of productive language, receptive language and maintenance of learned language. The first, on productive language, is also concerned with generalisation.

Garcia (1974) set out to identify the procedures and relations that lead to the acquisition of speech and its generalisations in students who previously lacked any conversational unit of speech. A girl of 12 years and young man of 18 years, both classified as profoundly retarded but not exhibiting any neurological damage were involved. Both had a small repertoire of words such as 'cookie' and 'candy'. They were to be taught a conversational sequence of three segments. In segment 1 a picture of an object (cut from a mail order catalogue) was displayed and the student had to ask 'What is this?' The teacher responded: 'This is a . . .; What do you see?' Student 'It's a . . .'. The teacher then asked 'Do you want the . . .?' and the student responded: 'Yes I do.' Teaching involved four responses:

1. The question ''What is that?'' was taught. The teacher showed the picture and waited for 10 seconds for a response and if it was not given modelled it for the student and went on to the next trial. Correct responses were reinforced and training continued until a preset response had been reached.

2 & 3. A similar procedure was followed to teach the answer to the experimenter's question 'This is a . . .; What do you see;' and the response 'Yes, I do.'

4. Here the full chain of responses was taught by bringing together 1–3 in the sequence devised to provide an example of conversational speech. In addition, testing of the learnt conversational unit was undertaken with different adults and in different settings.

Both students learnt the conversational sequences for four different pictures of objects though previously their speech had been essentially imitative. In addition, generalisation was found to questions from other individuals and in other settings. In many cases, however, generalisation of this kind might need to be programmed, i.e. the individuals and settings in which the teaching took place would need to be varied in order to ensure that the learned sequence was not used exclusively in one training setting with a single teacher.

It should also be added that a study of this sort provides a demonstration of what students who are profoundly retarded *can* achieve through use of individual behavioural teaching. It is clear, however, that the conversational unit is a highly artificial one and not one that would necessarily enable the person to function any more competently in his or her surroundings. At best we should view this as a powerful demonstration that even with low-functioning individuals with minimal conversational repertoires progress can be made. In order to go beyond such demonstrations, however, more flexible approaches leading to adaptive communication skills need to be evolved and we will turn to these later.

Garcia's demonstration emphasises productive speech, though clearly in this as in any other conversation sequence the individual is learning a receptive skill as well. McCuller and Salzberg (1984) dealt specifically with teaching receptive language to three adults who were profoundly retarded in a study of their ability to follow instruction. The three men involved ranged from 37 to 51 years of age and all had IQs below 10, though all were able to walk and feed themselves. The basic design was to teach the students to follow simple actions with objects, e.g. 'Pull yarn' or 'Grasp spoon'. The teacher gave the instruction and employed praise and food as reinforcers when a correct response was made. Physical prompts were employed where an incorrect response was made. These were faded by waiting for increasing durations of time before giving such assistance. Generalisation was tested by representing action-object combinations that had not been taught, e.g. in the above example it might be 'Grasp yarn'. All three men learnt to follow the action-object instruction and indeed generalised to novel combinations. However, the number of teaching trials to accomplish this was enormous, ranging from over 3,000 to over 5,500 trials. Nevertheless, it must be emphasised that the students were extremely profoundly retarded yet had learnt to follow a complex instruction and to do so under novel conditions.

At a simpler level of communication, receptive language teaching will usually entail learning to name objects. Welch and Pear (1980) study is of special interest in this respect since the students included Andy, a 9 year old boy with Down's Syndrome who was profoundly retarded (Mental Age (MA) = 2-2.5 years), and Cathy, a 14 year old girl functioning at a 2.5-3 year level who was cerebral palsied and had spastic quadriplegia. Though Cathy's receptive response was not verbal we will consider the results from her programme with those of Andy here.

An additional interest in this study is that the authors were not only concerned with receptive language in itself, but in the effect of the way in which the objects to be named were represented. Thus they used picture-cards, photographs and real objects. The majority of the items used were common household objects such as a fork, a magazine, etc. While Andy had to make a verbal naming response when shown an item, Cathy first made an observing response by pointing to the item for five seconds with her right arm then pointing to a Blissymbol representing the item. Basic operant procedures were employed and a teaching design which allowed a comparison of how far learning with items in a given seqeunce (e.g. pictures then real objects) affected generalisation of naming outside the situation.

Both Andy and Cathy successfully learnt receptive responding in their respective modalities, i.e. vocal and pointing to the Blissymbols. Both also showed generalisation of these responses to the natural environment. For Andy, however, this occurred equally whether initial training involved picture-cards, photographs or real objects. For Cathy, like other more able children taught in this study, teaching with real objects led to greater generalisation than when it had been carried out with pictures. Though not great, this did represent the first time that she had ever showed use of Blissymbols in the environment.

In the final study to be considered we will look at maintenance of learned communication, that is, endurance over time. Garcia and DeHaven (1980) note that there is very little information on long-term follow-up on the extent to which speech taught through language programmes is maintained. They report on the follow-up of a boy, John, who when 10 years of age participated in a study undertaken by DeHaven and Garcia (1974). At that time John lacked speech, was functioning at a 2 years 2 months level and was described as 'hyperactive'. At the time of the follow-up he was 16 years and his MA had advanced to 2 years 11 months. The authors summarise their findings:

> John did not maintain his generalized skill and the results of the present replication study are similar to those in the original research. In brief, continued training was effective in re-establishing the generalized speech usage but with much more training than was initially expected. Once a skill has been taught it is not, at least in John's case, easier to reinstate with the same training procedures. (p. 158)

This group of studies clearly show the applicability of standard behavioural procedures with children, young people and adults with profound retardation. Not only can productive and receptive language be taught, but quite complex generalisation can be established. Though maintenance of the original training and extent of generalisation has rarely been studied, the last piece of work offers a pessimistic view of the likelihood of communication skills learnt in this way maintaining without continued input. There is probably little doubt that if maintenance could be ensured then the behaviour would endure, but a demonstration of this sort does not actually take us to the point at which we have shown that flexible adaptive communication skills have been successfully taught.

Application of the behavioural model to people who are profoundly retarded has clearly demonstrated their capacity to communicate, but what steps do we take to go beyond these procedures to ensure that functional communication of the kind described in Chapter 3 in Volume 1 is learnt and spontaneously used? The overall criticism of tight programming of the sort described has been summarised by Rogers-Warren, Warren and Baer (1983): 'Most language intervention has been in the form of individualized training in specific structures of the linguistic system, including vocabulary, syntax, semantics, and to a very limited extent, pragmatic use (p. 240).

These and other authors have suggested ways in which language programming may be developed in order to ensure that children deficient in language learn communication skills that are truly functional. Before moving on to specific programmes that set out to meet this aim, we will summarise their position.

With respect to individuals with profound retardation, Rogers-Warren *et al.* (1983) point out that, as we have seen above, many learning trials are required for generalisation to take place. They suggest that this reflects an overemphasis on grammatical structures in their own right and insufficient consideration of the level of skill in social interaction required to enable the learner to use that linguistic structure: 'Establishing a comprehensive communication repertoire may require teaching both linguistic and social aspects of communication; however, few training programs specify training for anything except the structural aspects of language' (p. 244). While direct intervention increases the performance of linguistic behaviours, it may still engender artificiality through excessive prompting and the artificial time-phase of interactions between teacher and student.

These authors turn to the literature on mother-child interactions that we have reviewed in Chapter 3 in Volume 1. The importance of the natural social and communicative interchanges between mother and child in the construction of language is emphasised. Similarly, the extent to which impairments can disrupt or distort this flow (see Chapters 4–6 of Volume 1) are pointed out. In the light of the limitations on direct instruction, they suggest a more ecologically based approach to language teaching should be adopted. In such an approach the learner is seen as an active participant in interactions. First, the student must interact with the environment in order to provide a context in which communication can take place; secondly, the student must also interact with the teacher in this communicative context — though not necessarily verbally. The student has many options that enable participation including signalling attention, nonverbal responses and initiations, imitations and spontaneous verbal initiations and responses. These interchanges occur in a turntaking fashion with interest focused on the interaction. The process that goes on in such interactions is regarded as being akin to shaping in a behavioural programme. With respect to children who are retarded, Rogers-Warren *et al.* write:

> Several typical characteristics may impede or disrupt the natural process that supports language learning. First, if developmentally delayed children are less responsive, their lower rates of verbal and nonverbal imitations and responses reduce their caregivers' opportunities for teaching. To maintain a level of responding, mothers may use more direct speech, and thus non-directed or descriptive language. Lower levels of responsiveness may also make matching linguistic output to the child output more difficult, so that fine tuning present in normal mother-child interactions is less accurate with delayed children. Second, children who are not under instructional control (i.e. do not usually follow their mothers' instructions) may simply require more instructions. The relative difficulty of everyday tasks for the developmentally delayed child, and their typically shorter attention span, might both contribute to the need for additional instructions. If language teaching occurs more effectively and most frequently when there are no tasks to be accomplished and at the lead of the child, there may be fewer opportunities for teaching developmentally delayed children, who have greater difficulty and require more time to complete simple tasks and who interact less freely with the environment and their caregivers. Third, the same deficiencies that define developmental delay (difficulty in acquiring and generalizing new information, short-term memory constraints, and difficulty making small discriminations between similar stimuli) make the learning of languages in interactions more difficult than in the

normal child. If children do not easily discriminate fine cues for behavior, they must rely on more obvious cues. (p. 255)

In addition, insensitivity to social reinforcers may contribute to disruption of usual patterns of social interaction.

On the basis of these reviews, the authors suggest a 'conversation-based language learning model: . . . based on child-care giver interactions which must take into account the characteristics of mothers' behavior with their children, and the difference in responding between normal and atypical children' (p. 256). They go on to point out that all research evidence points towards mothers who have a high ability to adjust their own responding to variations in their child's behaviour. The teaching context they propose, therefore, is one in which the child is not simply a respondent but one in which he or she is interacting and learning to communicate pragmatically and is developing communicative strategies: 'The ideal teaching environment contains persons who do not respond naturally to the child's lowered responsiveness but seek to increase responsiveness without becoming unusually directive of the child's behavior' (p. 259). Thus:

> An ideal environment incorporates the characteristics of normal language-learning environments: appropriate language models presented when the child's attention is focussed on relevant aspects of the setting or interaction that the linguistic model describes; frequent opportunities to respond and appropriate cues for responding; and a supportive, responsive caregiver who follows the child's lead and consistently provides feedback about the child's attempts to communicate. (p. 260)

Because of the developmental delay, aspects of the situation may have to be made more obvious with respect to materials, motivation and context. Consistency is emphasised, but this must be dependent upon acute sensitivity to developments shown by the child. It is also important that some settings for working on language do not make other explicit curriculum demands; they should be playful but the setting must be clear to the child. Five recommendations are made: 1. Follow the child's lead. 2. Assume the child is trying to communicate and accommodate these attempts in some appropriate way. 3. Also make sure that you always respond in some way to the child's attempt to communicate whether through reinforcement or feedback. 4. When providing corrective feedback do so in a gentle positive way. 5. Talk with the child limiting instructions and directives.

Rogers-Warren *et al.* propose a major shift in the way that we approach language intervention with students who are language deficient. However, while their position has arisen from limitations that have emerged from evaluation of earlier behavioural approaches, it should not be taken that this implies a total rejection of those methods. Any worker with individuals who are profoundly retarded should be fully familiar with developing and implementing programmes that set out to teach syntactic or semantic aspects of language. The importance of the demonstrations reviewed above showing that extremely retarded people can learn language should not be under-emphasised. What we can envisage, however, is a continuum from situations in which such techniques are employed in a way that the students' ability to adapt through communication to their environment is enhanced, through to more flexible interactive teaching strategies of the kind just described.

With respect to students who are profoundly retarded and multiply impaired it is particularly important to keep this dimension in mind. With such individuals the lack of responsiveness, lowered instructional control, and psychological difficulties noted by Rogers-Warren *et al.* will mean that adjustment to the natural patterning of interactions that these authors propose as an ideal will press the teacher back into a careful consideration of several elements of the situation. These include presentation of stimuli, verbal and nonverbal, and systematic use of reinforcement. While realisation of a programme in such cases may look little different from earlier forms of direct intervention, the suggestion that teaching takes place in a meaningful communicative context must remain paramount if the failures of earlier programmes are not to be repeated.

Rogers-Warren *et al.'s* approach also brings to our attention a further feature of communicative interaction with people with profound retardation and multiple impairments. Most interactions do not take place in formal teaching situations but in everyday exchanges. Informal observation will show how finely tuned the response caregivers make to such students can be, how responses are delayed to give the person time to communicate, how cues are clearly presented and so on. The advice offered suggests a general strategy to be employed whenever a communicative context is established, not only in formal teaching settings.

It must be admitted, however, that general though the views just summarised have become during the past few years, there is as yet no comprehensive study of their application with people who are profoundly retarded. In order to provide any parallels to the strict operant studies reviewed above, we must at this point describe interventions that have tried to move decisively into the natural environment and teach communication in settings with real meanings to the participants. Such studies may be ranged on a continuum from those that attempt to apply in a natural setting specific techniques derived from operant approaches, to more global changes in social and physical aspects of the environment. For example, the target of reinforcing a communication made spontaneously by an individual in a living environment would represent the extension of a procedure from individual teaching methods to a natural setting. Introduction of material that should encourage interactions and hence communication, e.g. adding toys to an under-stimulating play room, would be an example of environmental modification. Again, in considering these approaches we are here concerned with the more able members of the population with which this book is concerned.

The introduction of a specific technique to facilitate communication can be illustrated by Halle, Marshall and Spradlin's (1979) application of a time-delay technique to increase language and facilitate its generalisation. They point out that staff often fail to recognise naturally occurring opportunities for teaching language because their own training has focused too specifically on the basic operant approaches described above. These authors worked in a setting in which no opportunities were provided for children to use language, i.e. at mealtime in the residential setting in which they lived. While all children were able to walk, most were classified as profoundly retarded. The basic procedure employed was as follows: At breakfast the child was called to the food counter. The target behaviour was defined as the child requesting his or her meal by using the word 'want' before and/or 'please' after any of the following words: 'tray', 'food', 'meal', 'eat'. The server held the tray with the food for 15 seconds (the time delay) until the child made the appropriate request. If this did not occur or was incorrect the tray was handed over at the end of this time. Failure by the child to make any appropriate request was followed by modelling plus the delay, i.e. at the end of 15 seconds the staff member modelled the request 'Tray please'. This was repeated at five-second intervals if the child did not respond and the tray was given to the child 15 seconds after the last model. If, however, the child made the request in response to the model, the tray was handed over.

Only one child learnt to make the request as a result of the time delay without modelling, while the addition of modelling succeeded with two more of the children. A fourth child required more intensive training. Three of the children had the opportunity to observe some of the other children learning the request and showed an immediate increase in requesting when the delay technique was etablished with them.

When requesting at breakfast had been established, the same procedure was introduced at lunchtime. Introduction of the time-delay procedure here led to immediate requesting by all children. When new servers were introduced at breakfast and at lunch and in a completely novel combination of new server at supper, good generalisation was shown for some, though not all, the children.

Halle *et al's* study shows that the introduction of specific procedures from behavioural teaching practice can enhance adaptive communication in the natural environment, even in children with profound retardation. It can be regarded as a highly structured example of Rogers-Warren *et al.*'s (1983) suggestions as to how adults can adjust their behaviour and activities to provide opportunities and time for children whose language is deficient.

Warren and Rogers-Warren (1983) also show how attention must be given to the actual environment as being conducive or otherwise to use of language and generalisation. In Halle *et al.*'s study there is a face validity to looking for generalisation at other mealtimes. Warren and Rogers-Warren employed the language programme devised by Guess, Sailor and Baer (1978) and described above with a group of children several of whom can be classified as profoundly retarded. They considered generalisation of noun learning to different settings. This was most extensive with respect to the classroom where teaching staff were responsive to language in contrast to non-teaching staff in some of the living units. In addition, relevance of the words learnt to settings also played a part, food-related words obviously being more likely to be used at mealtimes. They advocate, therefore, attention to adult behaviour in encouraging generalisation and to organisational features of the setting. They cite a study by VanBiervliet, Spangler and Marshall (1979) where a family-style dining arrangement was established for institutionalised children. Instead of collecting their food from the counter, it was put on the table and children had to pass the bowls to each other. This led to a large increase in verbal interactions among children and had the spin off of their eating more slowly.

All the above examples illustrate ways in which natural settings may be adjusted to increase the opportunity for language learning. Such an approach is also applicable to individuals who through physical impairment are unable to care for themselves. Ivancic, Reid, Iwata, Faw and Page (1981) draw attention to the usefulness of care routines in enhancing interactions between care staff and children. In this instance, the children were indeed both profoundly retarded and multiply impaired and we will describe them fully: Five profoundly retarded residents, ages

3 to 7 years, participated. All were multihandicapped, nonambulatory and dependent on staff for meeting basic care needs. Medical diagnosis of four children involved cerebral palsy with additional disorders including spina bifida, microcephaly, quadriplegia and hydrocephalus. The medical diagnosis for the fifth child included neuromuscular dysfunction due to cerebral atrophy and hydrocephalus. Three children received daily medication for seizure control. Each child had been recommended by centre professionals for training to increase sound production and imitation. Three children had notable deviations in speech mechanisms (e.g. cathedral palate). At the time of the study, none of the children made identifiable requests other than crying, none imitated sounds, and none followed any commands except for making intermittent eye contact when someone called their name. These particular residents were selected because they were the youngest and/or least vocal of the unit.

The staff involved in the study were direct care staff responsible for bathing and grooming the children. The setting chosen was the bathroom area of the children's living area and generalisation was assessed in an adjacent room. Four classes of staff behaviour were considered: 1. Any vocalisation directed towards the child (antecedent vocalisation). 2. Any vocalisation that described the resident's vocalisation (descriptive praise). 3. Imitation of the resident's vocalisations (sound imitation). 4. Vocalisations by staff prompting the child, e.g. 'Say: o-o-o' (sound prompt). Children's behaviour was recorded with respect to 'appropriate vocalisations', i.e. all vocalisations that were not piercingly loud or throaty, crying accompanied by a motor tantrum or patently involuntary sounds such as hiccuping. Appropriate vocalisations included single vowel sounds and consonant/vowel sounds.

The intervention was carried out by a supervisor who conducted initial in-service training with care staff in which the approach to language training was described and the value of, for example, staff vocalising described. This was followed by prompting the staff while dealing with the children, direct instructions and use of posters. Individual and group feedback was given. On all four categories of staff vocalisation a marked increase over a baseline assessment was shown and this was maintained over several months and generalised to the second setting. In addition, careful checks showed that there was no reduction in the cleanliness of the children or in how long it took to bathe and dress them. Thus, the introduction of the programme did not detract from the care role of the staff. The effect on the children was highly variable. Though one child showed a dramatic improvement in vocalising, the effect on the others was not consistent. As the authors note, however, the programme was only in effect for five months, and the procedures have not in the past been employed with individuals with such profound impairments and require further study.

This last study is specially important on three counts. First, it is one of the few that deals explicitly with individuals who are profoundly retarded and multiply impaired. Second, it reflects the convergence of two streams we have described in this chapter, i.e. the use of specific techniques such as modelling and imitation, and the need to undertake intervention in the environment in which the person lives and in naturally occurring social situations. Third, it represents an attempt at intervention which closely parallels the kind of situation normally occurring between parent and child that we have seen (Chapter 3 of Volume 1) to make such a significant contribution to the development of child language. A study undertaken at this level of communicative development also takes us back into the prerequisites of language development and intervention before individuals can enter typical language programmes. We now turn to this issue with special reference to early vocalisation and signalling behaviour and the link between cognitive prerequisites of language described in the previous chapter and language intervention.

The Prerequisites of Language

Prespeech

Later, with respect to choosing nonspeech modes of communication, we point out that early feeding difficulties are often predictive of subsequent speech problems. For this reason, dealing with feeding problems together with the encouragment of early vocalisation can be seen as the earliest phase of intervention in a comprehensive communication programme. Such intervention can be undertaken by a speech therapist, or by parents and teachers under the therapist's direct or written guidance. Warner (1981a) points out that feeding difficulties will often result from a wider pattern of neuromotor damage that also leads to spasticity, athetosis or hypotonia, and hence remediation will be part of a wider programme of physical therapy (see Chapter 5). She advocates that following detailed assessment, remediation will be directed to the development of posture, increasing or decreasing oral sensitivity, increasing tongue and lip control, developing acceptance of solid food, and the selection of feeding utensils to develop control of the mouth.

As noted, the neurological damage giving rise to eating difficulties will also affect speech production. Warner (1981b) emphasises that there can be no rigid approach to encouraging and developing early sound production. The child's own production abilities will be a guide to which sounds should be targeted. She notes the following possible levels of facilitation:

(i) imitation of vowel sounds and cadence;
(ii) facilitation of selected consonants either by eliciting the movement for sound or in imitation;
(iii) development of consonant vowel sounds;
(iv) imitation of words that encourage specific development of phonological approaches. Such developments lead into speech programmes with the characteristics noted in this chapter.

Pragmatic Functions and Social Interaction

The reaction against earlier attempts at behavioural intervention of the kind described above has been reinforced by our increasing understanding of the pragmatic nature of communication and its roots in social interaction. We described in some detail these aspects of language acquisition in Chapter 3 of Volume 1, and McLean and Snyder-McLean (1984) review them in relation to remedial language programmes. They suggest that the teacher of language will generate objectives that will involve communicative performatives of the following kind; '*Answering* (yes/no/ok); *Directing action* (help me/please/open up); *Directing attention* (look/big/oh-oh/meow); and *Greeting* (hi/bye-bye)' (p. 72). While these examples are concerned with early language, similar functions can be proposed for referencing and performative needs of older children. Thus, the pragmatic examples of language can be integrated with our knowledge of other dimensions of language as it increases in complexity and as the individual's needs become more complex. It is also necessary, they argue, that the individual learns how to conduct a discourse, i.e. to carry out normal and effective communication even though their language may be relatively primitive. A further implication of considerable importance in any consideration of individuals who are profoundly retarded is suggested by McLean and Snyder-McLean. This is, that we should also consider and target the nonlinguistic pragmatic aspects of communication, notably with respect to gesture. They point out how in earlier work they found adolescents who were severely retarded using only the most primitive gestures, e.g. an imperative consisting of holding out a glass to request more to drink. This repertoire they suggest should be expanded with special reference to nonfood-related requests (imperative function); directing the attention of others (declarative function); and responding to questions (answering function). It is their belief that higher levels of language can be attained if a non-linguistic repertoire of performatives of this sort is in place.

It is a short step from the position advocated above by McLean and Snyder-McLean to a further emphasis on the social context of language acquisition. These authors fully support the ecological position argued above. In achieving this they emphasise aspects of normal language acquisition described in some detail in Chapter 3 of Volume 1: 'These strategies include modifications of language addressed to children, including length reduction, complexity reduction, frequent repetition and paraphrasing' (p. 77). They also believe that more attention should be paid to the role of gaze and attending during teaching interactions concerned with language teaching. These strategies and those concerned with pragmatic function have been drawn together by McLean and Snyder-McLean (1985) in an outline of the approach they are advocating.

While the position described above will undoubtedly receive growing attention in the coming years, little has yet been published involving people who are profoundly retarded and multiply impaired. Coupe, Barton, Barber, Collins, Levy and Murphy (1985), however, have evolved an instrument that directly reflects the considerations underlying a pragmatic-interactive approach to language teaching. The Affective Communication Assessment provides an initial observational procedure that generates data that are intended to be used to identify the consistency and type of behaviours which might form the basis of intervention. Potentially communicative behaviours are identified as are the settings in which they are likely to occur. This permits the teacher to prepare and implement a consistent response within the student's daily routine. The context of such intervention draws explicitly on the available information on mother-child interactions. Seven aspects of the interaction are specified:

(i) Vocalisation by teacher, both in use of words (such as the child's name) and sounds.

(ii) Facial expression, e.g. smiling or frowning.

(iii) Physical proximity, i.e the teacher should be close to the student and in his or her visual field.

(iv) Eye contact and mutual regard: the student's head should be physically moved to ensure this if necessary.

(v) Physical contact: mutual touch with prompting of the child to touch if necessary.

(vi) Imitation of the child's sounds and facial expressions.

(vii) Turntaking, with the adult giving the child time to respond.

Several case studies using the assessment instrument and planning interventions on the basis of the information it produced are available.

Distress signalling is a special case of affective communication and Fraser and Ozols (1981) have examined the way in which crying, moaning and motor behaviour are interpreted by caregivers.

It will be noted that many of the procedures advocated parallel those developed by Ivancic *et al.* (1981) whose staff training approach could well be employed in implementing Affective Communication Assessment-based programmes. In complementary fashion, the use of such an assessment device in a care or other setting could be one way of ensuring that the actual interactions encouraged were based on sound assessment information. Given the somewhat disappointing oucome of Ivancic *et al.*'s study with respect to child behaviour, such an approach merits consideration.

In Chapter 2 we gave a general account of co-active intervention and its specific use in sensorimotor teaching. An approach to encourage communication through interaction has been derived from co-active intervention techniques (Chaper 3 of this volume). Sternberg and Owens (1985) interpret the Van Dijk procedure and present a programme for developing communication through interaction. Their starting point, in line with the developments in language programming described above, emphasises that meaningful communicative behaviour refers to the ability of the person to communicate in an interactive social context. Their starting point is the use of co-active techniques in order to encourage sensorimotor development as described in Chapter 3. Specifically they are concerned to teach two prelanguage accomplishments: (i) that the person can communicate; and (ii) that there are things to communicate about to people with whom communication is possible. As a result of moving the child through the social and sensorimotor developments by use of resonance, co-active movement and deferred imitation, what Sternberg and Owens refer to as 'natural gesture communication' will emerge. Such gestures are by definition self-developed and will represent what the person can do with an object (e.g. throwing motion for ball) or reference to the object (e.g. scooping motion with hand for 'spoon').

Sternberg, Pegnatore and Hill (1983) employed the approach described with four students who were profoundly retarded. This proved effective at the earliest level of the programme, i.e. the use of resonance to increase communicative awareness. Success in this aim and effective generalisation was demonstrated. Sternberg and Owens (1985) dealt with three young people who were profoundly retarded at stages beyond application of resonance. Again, it will be useful to characterise these people more fully: (1) was 18 years old and had arrested hydrocephaly and unco-ordinated movement as well as numerous behaviour disorders; (2) was a 13 year old with no major physical or sensory disabilities though did suffer from seizures and from tuberous sclerosis; (3) was a 22 year old man who was legally blind and suffered from seizures. Again, he showed behaviour disorders.

Sternberg and Owen's (1985) procedure was designed to elicit from each student a vocal or motor signal which would be used to indicate a desire to produce a co-active imitation behaviour. Such behaviour was taken as an indicator of a higher level of expressive communication than that expressive signalling accomplished during resonance levels of prelanguage communication.

> The following is a synopsis of the instructional procedure: The experimenter assumes a position in close proximity to but not in physical contact with the subject. The position assumed should be one that is easily observed by the subject. The experimenter should display a fine-motor or vocal signal that will be used to initiate a coactive imitation movement/position. The signal should then be followed immediately by the coactive movement position. The signal-to-coactive movement/position sequence should be shaped (using verbal and/or physical guidance prompts) until the subject consistently displays the fine-motor or vocal signal followed by self-initiation of the coactive movement/position. This self-initiation is done in order to effect the experimenter to follow the coactive imitation/movement position.

On the basis of observation, targets for teaching and co-active activities were selected. For example, for the first student the co-active activity was rolling a ball back and forth and a verbal 'buh' was used to initiate the activity. The intervention was carried out using behavioural techniques of the kind described elsewhere in this book. In phase 1 the teacher provided a repetitive signal while attempting to shape the signal from the student. Production of the signal was followed by the teacher adopting the co-active movement/position. In phase 2 the student had to produce both signal and co-active behaviour in sequence. In phase 3 the demand was production of this without any prior signal from the teacher.

The first student succeeded on all four phases, though the second and third students only reached criterion on phase 1. In effect, that meant that students (2) and (3) did learn to imitate the signal but never to chain it to the co-active behaviour. A further study by Sternberg *et al.* (1985) demonstrated the effectiveness of direct instruction in coactive imitation with individuals who were profoundly retarded and multiply impaired.

The upward extension of interaction-based programmes of the kind described by Sternberg and Owens and Coupe and her colleagues can be found in Carney *et al.*'s Social Skill Development assessment device also described in Chapter 7 of Volume 1. As in the Affective Communication Assessment, Carney *et al.* include touch as a programming objective, and an illustrative programme is presented — albeit of a relatively high level skill, i.e. naming people. Their programme extends into a second domain concerned with social interaction, namely social acceptability training. Here assessment of, and teaching objectives concerned with, physical appearance, appropriate movement, maintaining socially acceptable distances from people when interacting and other aspects of interaction are covered. With respect to both interaction and suitability, the authors note the need to tailor programmes to the level and nature of the person's additional impairments though specific programmes and directions for this are not given.

Cognition

We have described in some detail the evidence that points to the fact that there are important cognitive prerequisites to language development (Volume 1, Chapter 3). We have also indicated that this holds in the case of people with profound retardation (Volume 1, Chapter 8). Programming for language development also, therefore, requires consideration of teaching appropriate cognitive prerequisites. Kahn (1984) suggests that the failure of most language teaching based upon operant methods results from the fact that students 'had been taught only to respond on cue and were not cognitively ready to use referential speech' (p. 15).

We have already reviewed the evidence produced by Kahn (1975) showing that this cognitive influence is reflected in the fact that Stage VI of sensorimotor functioning has to be achieved for spoken language to emerge. He writes:

If, as these findings seem to indicate, the cognitive structures of Stage 6 of Piaget's sensorimotor period must develop before the initial use of productive speech, then planning for productive oral language development training of nonverbal profoundly retarded children should begin with an assessment of their cognitive level. Children who are at Stage 6 can reasonably be expected to begin learning oral language skills. (Kahn 1975 p. 16)

We have already seen that the possibility of such a cognitive assessment is feasible with children who are profoundly retarded (Volume 1, Chapter 7) and that where they are below Stage VI suitable sensorimotor training methods can be devised (Chapter 3). Thus, the training of cognition in the sensorimotor part of the curriculum can be seen both as an end in its own right leading to an increased understanding of the world, *and* as contributing to the communication curriculum in that it trains prerequisite skills relevant to that domain.

In view of the dual function of sensorimotor training and the fact that one aspect has been dealt with in the previous chapter, there is little to add with respect to sensorimotor teaching and communication. Such teaching will, in any comprehensive curriculum, span the full curricular range. Any special focus on communication prerequisites will be on the development of the object concept, means-end behaviour and vocal imitation. On achieving a given criterion on these scales, the student will move into a more advanced phase of language training involving single words and word combinations. We say 'more advanced' because, of course, work will have been going on on teaching interactions in parallel to sensorimotor teaching. The choice of a specific language programme approach will reflect decisions made in the light of issues raised in the first section of this chapter.

In order to illustrate the general course of events in evolving a programme that takes us from sensorimotor development into a language programme we will briefly summarise a report by Kahn (1984) involving 24 children with profound retardation, Chronological Ages (CAs) between 3 and 10 years. All were free of sensory handicaps though some measure of physical impairment is suggested by the comment that 'the children were all able to control at least one arm well enough to perform the object permanence and means-end tasks required of them' (p. 17). The children were assessed on the Uzgiris-Hunt Scales, a developmental scale, and Bricker, Dennison and Bricker's (1976) prelinguistic and linguistic assessment. The children were pretested and then retested at various times after implementation of the programme.

Three groups of eight children took part. One group received object concept training followed by language teaching, the second, means-end training then language training and the third group, only language training. All children in the object concept group achieved the sensorimotor objectives and five achieved some of the language training goals. Six children in the means-end group achieved these objectives and all six made progress in the language programme. None of the children in the language programme only group showed progress in this area and none showed any cognitive improvement. Maintenance of these gains for the training was good and some of the children in both groups showed evidence of generalisation.

With entry into a formal language programme at Sensorimotor Stage VI, we also enter the preoperational stage and the areas of the cognitive curriculum described in the preceding chapter, particularly with reference to the work of Lavatelli (1970a, b). In this, classification, number, measurement, space, seriation, etc. will be taught. Lavatelli emphasises that in teaching these cognitive skills every opportunity should be taken to use the situation to encourage verbalisation of the relations involved in the task.

With respect to language teaching with people with mental handicap, this position has been elaborated by Miller and Yoder (1972; 1974). In Chapter 3 of Volume 1 we described the theoretical background to their approach in which the person's understanding of the world is seen to entail the encoding of this experience in words that are organised syntactically. In Table 3.1 of that chapter, relations and functions at the one- and two-word levels are listed. These describe functions such as existence of an object, the agent of an action, the object of an action and so on. Miller and Yoder emphasise two points. First, that at least in the early stages of language development understanding of these relations precedes the development of the appropriate syntactic structures. Second, that the events that occur which exhibit these relations and which are used in teaching should come from the actual world of the person. Taken together this would mean that an understanding of 'pat pussy' would be required before teaching this action-object relation *and* that there would have to be a cat in the person's home that was patted. In addition, this frequency of occurrence is going to reflect the communicative value of the utterance for the child, a fact that links this approach to the broader interactional context we described earlier. In selecting content for language teaching, Miller and Yoder suggest that the chosen teaching sequence should reflect the frequency of occurrence of appropriate events in the individual child's world, and should also draw on the picture of normal language development which is given in Table 3.1. It must be emphasised, however, within the stages listed there are no rigid sequences and children do show individual differences.

At a general level, Miller and Yoder see the language content of Table 3.1 as providing the format for a language programme. The approach emphasises that since cognition cannot be directly manipulated, it is through environmental structuring that language can be enhanced: 'By pairing explicit environmental experiences with their linguistic referent, the child will note these relations and begin to express them' (Miller and Yoder 1974, p. 520). As these authors point out, behavioural programmes have typically emphasised the relational aspect without reference to the actual environment. McCuller and Salzberg's (1984) study reviewed above exemplifies this. Here arbitrarily selected objects and in general arbitrary relations (e.g. push alligator) were employed in an action-object context. Thus the linguistic and the environmental experiences must be paired in the teaching context.

The training sequence suggested by Miller and Yoder follows a five-step course. First, the person should be exposed to the words that describe the particular event. For example, the teacher would say and demonstrate 'push ball'. No verbal response would be required from the student. Second, the teacher must establish that the student understands the words employed to mark the event. Third, the teacher pairs words and events and teaches imitative responses. Fourth, fade the model for imitation and encourage spontaneous expression of the event. Fifth, encourage expression of the relation by fading the action-object sequence. Thus, the student would say 'push ball' and this would become the reinforcement for that event.

While Miller and Yoder emphasise working on a single event-language pairing to start with, it should be in mind that generalisation is likely to be enhanced by teaching with sufficient exemplars as early as possible in the programme. Following expression of a particular relation in a variety of settings, these authors then suggest that the particular function be expanded. A final point they emphasise is that in such teaching situations the language employed by the teacher should be structured to maximise the student's comprehension. This can involve simplification and emphasis of the kind we have seen parents spontaneously make in order to communicate with young children.

As with our discussion of cognitive teaching, we have moved appreciably up the ability range and made numerous assumptions about the degree to which the student has additional impairments. As Kiernan (1985) points out, however, studies of severely, let alone profoundly, retarded students undertaken on language teaching in the preoperational period hardly exist. A major gap in this area must be noted to which both teachers and research workers need to pay considerable attention. Nevertheless, developmentally many students will be at a level suitable for entry into the programme envisaged by Miller and Yoder and lesser impairments will not necessarily preclude this. However, we know that even where Sensorimotor Stage VI functioning has been achieved and the social basis for communication evolved, there will be individuals in this population for whom entry into a *verbal* language programme of the sort described here will be extremely problematical. We will shortly turn to these problems, and to the use of non-oral techniques. First, however, we will briefly deal with the somewhat paradoxical fact that some people with profound mental retardation do exhibit vocalisation that we might wish to eliminate.

Eliminating Inappropriate Vocalisation

The use of speech to communicate implies that it is appropriate to the context in which it is uttered. This appropriateness relates both to what has been said by another person and to the objects and events that are to be commented on. There are occasions when, despite showing quite sophisticated levels of syntax and vocabulary, some individuals' speech is not related to the communicative demands and conventions of the situation and intervention is called for. Reports in the literature have dealt with two major classes of inappropriate speech, echoism and speech unrelated to environmental inputs. Here we summarise some studies that deal with these classes of inappropriate speech in individuals with profound retardation and multiple impairments in order to illustrate the use of systematic, behavioural approaches to these problems.

Echoism

Echoism is the repetition by an individual of a word, phrase or sentence previously heard, often repeated several times. The imitation can be immediate or deferred. Ausman and Gaddy (1974) dealt with echoism in a functionally blind young woman of 17 years described as 'severely retarded' though no further details are given. Her verbal behaviour bears some resemblance to that occurring in nonretarded blind people noted in Volume 1, Chapter 4:

> She was able to repeat entire commercials, whole sentences of which she had previously heard spoken, and sing entire songs. However, she was completely unable to make appropriate responses to questions. Instead, she would repeat the question. She did not initiate appropriate conversation, referred to herself in the second person, and did not make requests. (p. 20).

The procedure adopted was a relatively simple one. Two teachers sat with the woman. The first asked a question softly then answered it in a louder voice. If she responded with an appropriate answer she was reinforced. If she did not respond, the second teacher repeated the question softly. Using this technique her appropriate, nonecholalic replies increased virtually to 100 per cent. A formal evaluation of generalisation was undertaken, but the authors report that outside the training session she then asked for items she wanted, responded appropriately to questions and generalised to many questions not included in her training.

Schreibman and Carr (1978) worked with two children, one of whom was profoundly retarded, though no additional impairments are reported. Though having some expressive and comprehensive language, the 15 year old girl always responded echoically to questions and had never been heard to say 'I don't know'. A verbal prompt-fading procedure was used to teach this last response. The teacher would ask a question followed by 'I don't know', e.g. 'How do trucks run? — I don't know', which would be echoed by the girl. This would be reinforced and the 'I don't know' progressively faded until the child said this herself without the model. In phase 2, questions to which she did have an answer (e.g. 'What's your name?') were interspersed in order that she should discriminate answerable from nonanswerable questions. In phase 3, reinforcement was considerably reduced.

The study showed that echolalic responding in this situation could be eliminated and good generalisation was shown. The girl did continue to answer questions she knew, showing that she was able to discriminate the two classes of question.

While both studies noted concentrated on the traditional one-to-one type of behavioural teaching, it is interesting to note that Halle *et al.*'s (1979) study reports that two of the children with profound retardation in the time-delay programme were echolalic. We may infer that the use of this technique in a free environmental situation can encourage speech in such children, though no information is given on whether echolalic speech was reduced or eliminated.

In contrast, inappropriate speech may be nonecholalic but may be unrelated in a discernible way to the immediate environmental experience. Barton (1970) describes a programme undertaken with an 11 year old boy classified as profoundly retarded with some physical impairment (he was quadriplegic but still able to walk clumsily) but no sensory impairment. She describes his speech in the following way:

Simon's speech was clearly articulated and his vocabulary large; however, much of what he said was quite inappropriate. He frequently perseverated with one response. When asked questions about magazine pictures, many of his responses appeared to be random and unconnected with the picture; he responded to even simple questions with advertising jingles and other inappropriate phases. Thus, for example, on one occasion he asked for a pencil, but when asked why, he replied 'to keep my shirt clean'. (p. 300)

Barton's programme aimed to teach appropriate answers to questions about mail-order catalogue pictures. The procedure was as follows: The teacher showed a picture to Simon who asked one of two questions of the general form — Question 1: Who, what, where is (that, doing ____)? or Question 2: What, where (is, are) he, she, it, they (doing, having, playing, etc.) (here, there, on, in the ____)? Responses were defined as appropriate, and reinforced; inappropriate, in which case time-out was employed, i.e. the teacher covered the pictures with her arms and turned away for 10 seconds; or negative, e.g. no response, in which case this was ignored and the teacher progressed to the next item. Generalisation testing was carried out with novel pictures and also a number of general conversational questions, e.g. 'Do you go to school?'

The result of the reinforcement and time-out procedures were that appropriate responding dramatically increased as inappropriate responding declined. The generalisation results were less impressive, though in the direction of increased appropriateness. While this study is again limited to the conventional one-to-one format, it points towards the possibility of eliminating inappropriate speech in the natural environment by ensuring that such speech is dealt with by a clear contingency such as time-out and that this kind of contingency is discriminated from positive reinforcement. This consistency should extend across individuals and environments if such a programme is to be fully effective.

Nonspeech Communication

The marked developments that have taken place in the use of nonspeech communication techniques in the field of mental handicap generally are of special relevance and interest to those concerned with people who are profoundly retarded and have additional impairments. Shane (1981) defines a nonspeech communication technique as a 'system or device that enhances a non-speaking person's current communication abilities' (p. 392). He distinguishes between communication prostheses and manual systems. The former include both electronic and nonelectronic communication aids and the latter manual signing systems (briefly reviewed by Kiernan 1983). In schools catering for children with mental handicap in England, 80 per cent have introduced some form of nonspeech communication systems (Jones, Reid and Kiernan 1982; Kiernan, Reid and Jones 1982). In the USA, Fristoe and Lloyd (1978) report a similar dramatic growth since 1972.

As Kiernan (1983) points out, this movement has been predominantly practitioner-led with research supporting the usefulness of the techniques. Light, Remington and Porter (1982) note that research justifies the conclusion that there 'seem to be good grounds, both theoretical and empirical, for giving consideration to alternatives to speech for certain types of severely handicapped children' (p. 223). It is not our intention here to pursue theoretical and experimental aspects of the body of research that has been generated over the past decade. The interested reader should turn to Kiernan (1983) and Remington and Light (1983) for this information. Here we are more concerned with the process of selection of nonspeech techniques for individual children and the implementation of different approaches. The former issue is of particular importance since several studies show that the initial selection of a particular system for a given group of children is often extremely haphazard. Surveys by Fristoe and Lloyd (1978) and Goodman, Wilson and Bornstein (1978) point to the fact that the main reason for selection of a given system is familiarity with it, rather than any careful assessment of the range of possible systems and their individual appropriateness for a given person. The authors of the former study comment on 'a lack of sophistication on the part of users with regard to non-speech communication systems' (p. 99). As an extreme example they describe an attempt to teach finger spelling to individuals with severe and profound retardation despite the fact that such learning would have to be based on rote learning and would require finer motor co-ordination than would be required to express the same meanings through simple signs.

Similarly, practitioners have often used only the most rough and ready criteria in electing a person to nonspeech communication and deciding whether this has been successful or otherwise. Fristoe and Lloyd (1978) state that selection criteria are usually global and do not take all relevant information into account, e.g. 'she is fifteen years old and with no useful spoken vocabulary'. With respect to deciding when failure has occurred, Goodman *et al.* (1978) show that practitioners would persist for varying periods of time, on average eight months, though some continued for 18 months. On deciding the chosen approach had failed, 46 per cent would attempt to introduce communication boards, 9 per cent would go back to speech programmes, and 28 per cent would not attempt anything further.

We have seen in the first part of this chapter that spoken language is a realistic aim for some people who are profoundly retarded even where, in addition, there are other impairments. How, though, do we set about determining that because of delay in the development of spoken language and in the face of additional impairments the time to consider electing a person to a non-oral communication programme has come? How, having made this decision, do we select a particular system or device?

There is as yet no properly evaluated system by which such decisions can be guided. However, it is clear that the choice to adopt a nonspeech communication system will reflect conclusions about the person drawn from the range of assessments described in these volumes, and an evaluation of the situations in which communication is a priority for that person. Failure to develop spoken language will reflect not only developmental factors related to an understanding of the world, but also the influence of sensory and physical impairments which we have already seen influence the course of language development in children who are not generally intellectually impaired (Chapters 4–6 of Volume 1). A detailed consideration of the totality of this information will lead us to a consideration of whether to elect for non-oral communication and the form this should take. How might we guide our decision-making?

Shane and Bashir (1980) evolved during the course of their clinical work what they refer to as an 'election-selection decision making matrix' which aims to provide answers to these questions. Though this can be employed as a formal assessment technique, it is more likely in a clinical setting to be used to guide assessment in a less formal way as an aid to coming to these decisions. We will here, therefore, summarise the main factors that these authors take into account rather than reproducing their specific procedure. The interested reader can find this in the article cited above (Shane and Bashir 1980) and in Shane (1981) and Ferrier and Shane (1983).

In making the initial choice as to whether the persons should be introduced to a nonspeech communication system, information from a variety of assessments will be required. It is important to note that this information will not have been gathered entirely with this aim in mind. The comprehensive approach to cognitive, physical and sensory assessment presented in these volumes as a basis for all aspects of curriculum will provide much of what is relevant. However, this information will require interpretation in the wider context of the person's life in order to establish its implications for effective communication.

Shane (1981) proposes a variety of factors that should be taken into account:

(i)   Presence of 'High-risk Condition': Surveys of language development show that mental handicap is one such condition and that poor speech development is associated with the condition. This state of affairs is even more apparent in people with profound retardation and is accentuated when additional impairments are present. In Shane's terms, then, individuals who are regarded as profoundly retarded with multiple impairments must be judged as such a high-risk group and this will be one factor in considering them for selection for nonspeech communication training.

(ii)   Oral Reflex Factors: The persistence of primitive oral reflexes will suggest damage to the person's central nervous system and will be reflected in persistence of rooting, suckle/swallow and bite reflexes, as well as an overactive gag reflex. Shane suggests that this particular factor is unique in deciding to elect for nonspeech communication as in isolation this is a sufficient factor for making the decision. No other criterion, he suggests, has such a strong singular influence. He does, however, emphasise the importance of careful assessment by pointing out that many factors related to bodily state, position, method and time of elicitation are important. It can be added that remediation of abnormal oral reflexes can in time change the overall picture with respect to this factor.

(iii)   Laryngeal Blocking: This is often charcteristic of people with cerebral palsy and results in the cessation of sound during the attempt to speak. Again, this failure is regarded as a good predictor of oral speech.

(iv)   Eating Problems: Shane reviews studies indicating that early feeding problems are predictive of later speech difficulties 'because they suggest the presence of neuromotor involvement of the oral structures. Furthermore, in cases where neuromotor involvement is uncertain, eating behavior, past and present, is suggestive of neuromotor compromise' (p. 397).

Assessment of feeding will point to deviant or pathological patterns including jaw-thrusting, tongue-thrusting, tonic bite reflex, lip retraction, tongue retraction and nasal pharyngeal reflex.

Points (ii)–(iv) above are likely to present in many people with profound retardation with neurological damage and particularly in the least able within this group. Confirmatory motor information that such damage exists and that speech will be influenced will come from the presence of cerebral palsy, abnormal vocal production consisting mainly of vowel sounds, undifferentiated or absence of speech sounds and excessive drooling.

(v)   Cognition: Shane's suggestion with respect to the development of understanding emerges directly from the literature on the relation between sensorimotor development and the emergence of language that we have reviewed earlier in this chapter and in Chapters 3 and 8 of Volume 1. Election to a non-oral communication system, it is argued, is equally dependent upon the development of cognition, specifically on acquisition of Sensorimotor Stage V as indicated on one of the instruments reviewed in Chapter 7 of Volume 1. Alternatively, an MA of 18 months might be taken as sufficient indication of readiness, though here it must be borne in mind that such a global indication might be arrived at with relatively weak achievements in highly relevant areas of cognition.

(vi)   Comprehension-Production Discrepancy: Within the range defining profound retardation that we have adopted, a marked discrepancy between production and comprehension ability is not likely. Within the developmental range, however, it is possible that comprehension at an 18 to 36 month level may have outstripped production. This will indicate that one important facet of language development has emerged and that failure of production suggests consideration of a nonspeech system to enhance expression and narrow the gap.

(vii)   Imitation: Though the role of imitation in language acquisition in natural situations is unclear, its value in initiating successful language training has been suggested in several behavioural studies. Shane suggests that a failure in the development of vocal imitation, particularly following sustained intervention, again points to a nonspeech system. In view of the failure in the development of imitation in people with profound retardation, this should be regarded as an important factor within the overall context of assessing cognition.

(viii)   Previous Intervention: With respect to imitation we noted that its failure to develop should be considered *after* an attempt to teach the ability. This consideration can be extended to take into account language intervention generally. Spoken language will always be the first choice for any individual and for many will have been attempted for some time. Shane writes that: 'The occurence of previous therapy, the nature of the intervention, and the individual's response (and perhaps rate of response) to that therapy must all be considered. If no previous therapy has been tried, then one could decide to delay introduction of an augmentative communication system until an approach has been tried' (p. 402). For individuals functioning below the appropriate level of sensorimotor development, of course, the therapy is likely to have been directed to improvement in oral functioning, sound production and feeding, while teaching will have taken the form of encouraging patterns of interaction that underlie more advanced communication. It would only be after sustained work and limited progress in these areas against a background of advancing cognition and perhaps comprehension that we would embark on a nonspeech system.

(ix) The Environment: We have emphasised above the importance of the individual's environment in considering language programmes. With reference to a nonspeech system, Shane argues that environmental factors must be taken into account in making the decision on whether to adopt such an intervention. Significant persons in the individual's life should be consulted as their co-operation is critical to the implementation and success of the approach adopted.

The factors outlined by Shane should be treated as guidelines to help in coming to a decision. Two factors, CA and emotional influences, have beem omitted as not obviously applicable to individuals with profound retardation and multiple impairment. They clearly entail interdisciplinary assessment involving teacher, speech therapist and physiotherapist and possibly a psychologist. For any given individual and situation they will have different weights and it has not been shown that the rigid application of these criteria is essential or feasible. Ferrier and Shane (1983) show how the procedures can be employed using a case history approach, as well as applying the system to individuals who are profoundly retarded with additional impairments.

The decision to elect for a nonspeech communication system leads us on to choosing between an aided or unaided system and selecting an appropriate system from among the options. Kiernan (1985) has recently summarised the main systems in both these categories and here we will simply list them without further description: With respect to sign languages and systems he noted: British Sign Language (BSL), American Sign Language (ASL), Signed English, British Sign Language-Makaton Vocabulary (BSL-M), Paget Gorman Signed Speech (PGSS), Amerind, and Finger Spelling. To these we can add the Australian Sign Language which is derived from BSL. With respect to aided systems, Kiernan notes: Communication boards, Graphic symbol systems, Blissymbolics, Rebus Systems, Sigsymbols, Premackese and word cards. The choice of one or more of these systems for both receptive and expressive communication will have to be made on the basis of individual considerations, and the second part of Shane and Bashir's (1980) system moves from election to selection. Here the significant factors that need to be taken into account relate to neuromuscular involvement, portability of the system, imitation skill level, rate of acquisition, preference towards pictures, gestural orientation and environmental considerations:

(i)   Neuromotor: While vocal tract involvement influenced election to a non-oral system, upper limb involvement will here be an important consideration. Where gross and fine movement is seriously impaired this will preclude effective use of manual signs and gestures as well as finger spelling. This difficulty is particularly likely to manifest itself in individuals with cerebral palsy. It should be added that even where specific neuromotor damage does not affect actual formation of individual signs, deficits in the ability to plan sequences of movement can reduce the effectiveness of signing as an expressive medium.

(ii)   Portability: Where an aided system is selected, its portability becomes a significant factor whether it has to be transported by the student or the caregivers.

(iii)   Response Rate: Where the option remains open as to whether a manual or aided system is employed, Shane suggests taking the differential rate of acquiring communicative skills into account. Since there is no research bearing on this point, this will be a matter of determining rate for an individual.

(iv)   Picture Orientation: This somewhat vague term is used by Shane to describe the individual who spontaneously uses pictures to communicate with and would benefit from a prosthesis with pictorial content.

(v)   Gesture Orientation: We have seen how hearing-impaired children evolve their own gestural communication systems (Volume 1, Chapter 5). Assuming motor abilities permit, then, a spontaneous use of gestures weighs on the side of a manual communication system.

(vi)   Environment: Learning a communication system that is only usable in a single environment, e.g. a school classroom, is clearly of limited value. Use of manual systems typically do not permit integration into the wider speaking community where sign languages are not known. Shane suggests that 'The use of a communication prosthesis might allow more social interaction since the written word or pictures are generally comprehensible. Shane suggests that clients, aware of this advantage, have requested such systems even for children who can sign in order to increase their ability to communicate with nonsigners. Again, consultation with significant people in the person's environment is essential.

(vii)   Imitation: Shane considers motor imitation as a prerequisite for signing. Typically such imitation will be of a visual configuration though imitation of a tacitly perceived model of the teacher's hand shape is feasible as will be seen later in relation to Wilson's (1983) study. Both methods could, of course, be employed with a shaping technique in which the sign is modelled for the student's hand.

Both Kiernan (1985) and Shane (1981) emphasise the individual nature of the decision-making for any given person. Though the factors to be taken into consideration with respect to election and selection are the basic concerns with regard to people with profound retardation and multiple handicap, they are by no means all embracing and complex interactions between them might influence our choice. With respect to the prerequisites for successful utilisation of communication boards, for example, McDonald (1976) suggests that the person must be able to attend to visual stimuli, to store and recall meanings associated with pictures and drawings, to physically indicate a picture and so on. Failure with respect to any such ability, if it has not precluded eventual choice of the device, might lead into programmes to teach such prerequisites in their own right. With respect to interactions, good prognosis with respect to motor development might influence choice, the initial selection taking into account possible improvement in this respect. The research reviewed by Kiernan (1985) does not at present bear in any direct way on such individual decisions however much it might affect general improvements in nonspeech communicative systems themselves.

Manual Signing

Having opted for a manual sign system, there are further considerations related to (i) method of teaching; (ii) choice of 'words'; (iii) maintenance and generalisation; and (iv) choice of system.

Teaching has typically been reported as being behavioural in approach. Kohl, Fundakowski, Menchetti and Coleman (1977), for example, employed two major phases, training of imitation of signs and then teaching expressive sign production involving manual labelling of objects and actions. In both phases physical prompting or hand-shaping is used, with, if necessary, an error correction procedure. Presentation of model or object/action would proceed by ensuring an attending response and, of course, reinforcement would follow a correct production of the sign. In parallel it is usually urged that the teacher says the appropriate word when presenting the sign, and Kohl *et al.* urge that signs should be faded if the person starts to produce the words verbally. Similarly, the teacher can say the word when the student produces the correct sign. Both PGGS and Signed English permit parallel production of signs and words as Kiernan (1985) points out.

Working in part with adults who were profoundly retarded, though with no additional impairments, Duker and Morsink (1984) described a behavioural training procedure based on the technique of transfer of stimulus control. Initially the teacher presents the object to be signed saying its name and signing at the same time. Failure to sign was followed by the progressive introduction of physical guidance and then fading of the guidance as signing developed. Following a sequence of correct responses, the teacher would stop signing the object, only giving the word for it. A similar procedure using pictures instead of words was also employed, i.e. the objective was to teach signing to the picture rather than the word. Both procedures proved successful within the limited context in which they were employed.

The choice of words and word combinations should be informed by the same considerations as those raised by Rogers-Warren and her colleagues and noted in the previous section on spoken language. The choice should be determined by the environmental demands which the individual encounters and not be arbitrary. The ability to use them should enhance adaptation to the world about. Developmentally, the language models should be at the limit of the student's expressive capacity. Kiernan (1985) emphasises the need to match the teacher's input of sign and speech, drawing the student on to increased vocabulary and syntax complexity. Elsewhere (Kiernan 1984) suggests that Signed English based on BSL should be developed on the main manual communication system for people with mental handicap, with Makaton being phased out and consideration given to phasing out PGSS. The need to maintain and generalisation of the learned signing would entail similar procedures to those involved in the teaching of spoken language. Techniques of the sort developed by Halle *et al.* are clearly directly applicable to a signing programme.

Aided Communication

While by definition manual signing is realised through a single means, aided communication comes in a variety of forms that is ever expanding as technology advances. The aided device may range from a communication board with pictures, symbols or words, through to equipment that employs speech synthesizers. The central concern, having elected for an aided device, however, is how in response terms the student is to communicate. Vanderheiden (1976) points out that this must not only be within the capabilities of the person, but must also be the most advantageous to them. He goes on to show that most methods involve variations on *scanning, encoding,* and *direct selection.*

Scanning involves the presentation, one by one, of the pictures, symbols or words and the student indicates when the recipient of the communication has chosen the required item. For example, the recipient might point to each of a series of pictures until the person indicates the chosen item has been selected. This indication can be verbal or gestural. Encoding is a more complex activity. The student here combines two or more differentiated responses to indicate the picture, word or letter. For example, in an array of pictures mounted chessboard fashion in rows and columns an indication of row number and column number would define the particular picture chosen. Again, the way this is indicated is flexible but this method is more abstract than scanning or direct selection and is liable to be problematical for young children and for those with cognitive impairments. Direct selection is the most straightforward and common approach where gesture or some form of pointing is employed to indicate the picture, symbol or word.

All three methods can be realised through a variety of means from simple finger pointing through to complex selection effected through use of a microprocessor. Vanderheiden (1976) describes four methods of realisation which he refers to as: (i) fundamental; (ii) simple electronic; (iii) independent, i.e. with permanent record of communication but not portable; (iv) independent *and* portable. Despite the upward progression implied in (i) to (iv), not all devices are applicable to differing ability groups. For those who cannot read and are at the picture or symbol level or who can only communicate at a one to two word level, it is the more basic systems with which we are concerned. Clearly, people with profound retardation and multiple impairments come within this category and we shall therefore concentrate here on systems employing pictures and symbols and consider fundamental techniques that permit scanning and direct indication.

Providing that there is one single controllable movement, then scanning is potentially applicable. Switches can be operated by almost any part of the body and failing this, breath-operated switches can be employed. Sequential scanning can be carried out with a linear array of pictures or symbols or they can be organised in a circle with scanning proceeding anti-clockwise or clockwise. Here only a limited vocabulary can be employed because of restriction on number of items and the technique demands a recipient of the communication to point or move a physical indicator.

With direct selection the communicator him or herself indicates the required picture or symbol. This is the simplest method and is particularly applicable to people with mental handicap who have sufficient motor control to make the selection.

The aided communication devices that can be employed using the scanning and direct selection methods are numerous and are described and illustrated at length in Vanderheiden and Grilley (1976). The available devices will, however, continue to expand in numbers and sophistication, though with a consequent increase in costs. Lloyd and Karlan (1984) summarise the position with respect to technological advances as follows:

The rapid progress in microcomputer technology and recent developments in rehabilitation engineering are already being felt. Earlier problems with graphic non-speech symbols such as their storage, retrieval, reproduction in each message, etc. have been substantially reduced by the graphics capabilities of today's microcomputer. In addition, rehabilitation engineering has reached the point that in theory, and almost completely in practice, even the most severely physically handicapped individual can have access to and operate a microcomputer. The issue before us now is how to translate this general progress into progress for the mentally handicapped individuals. Very basic approaches to training retarded individuals to use, however simply, microcomputers will need to be developed and evaluated; the software to do this training using the computer itself will have to be identified and adapted and developed. The hard tasks are ahead. (p. 15)

While we should have every expectation that people who are profoundly retarded and multiply impaired will benefit from these important advances, the reality of the present situation is that cheaper and more basic devices will continue to be used for some time to come. In the following section we describe some studies that have been undertaken with such people, first with respect to manual signing and then with regard to aided communication devices, particularly communication boards and the use of Blissymbols.

Using Manual Signing

Two studies involving profoundly retarded adults, some with hearing impairment, illustrate many of the general points made in this chapter regarding the ecological context of language teaching generally, and the specific requirements for entering a manual communication programme. Faw, Reid, Schepis, Fitzgerald and Welty (1981) set out to investigate and evaluate a programme for involving residential staff in developing and maintaining manual sign language skills in a group of people who were profoundly retarded. The six people came within this category both in intellectual development and adaptive behaviour and two were legally deaf. All had received vocal language teaching without success.

Nine manual signs were targeted, selected for their relevance to adaptive functioning in the living unit. Prior to implementation of the programme, staff received appropriate in-service training. Group training of residents consisted of the students sitting in a semi-circle around a primary trainer who provided instructions, modelled and gave feedback. The secondary trainer prompted individuals who gave inadequate responses. Two steps were employed in the programme. First, a picture of a target sign was held up with the question 'What is the sign for . . .?' For residents who did not give the appropriate sign, individual training within the group followed.

While learning of the signs for the nine target words was successfully achieved, there was no change in signing (or vocalising) by students on the living unit itself. Generalisation to actual objects from the pictures was then considered, as it was thought that such generalisation would be necessary if extension to staff interactions about objects was to occur. For four of the five students, signing for real objects was very limited and specific training was therefore introduced. Generalisation to staff was considered in structured interactions in which staff invited signing to specific objects on the ward. While signing did increase in these structured interactions, there was no increase in signing in free interactions.

This study in many ways appears to repeat the mistakes of earlier behavioural work in the field of spoken language teaching and led Schepis, Reid, Fitzgerald, Faw, van den Pol and Welty (1982) to approach the problem in a more ecological manner. This study employed incidental teaching procedures utilising naturally occurring interactions between clients and caregivers as a format to increase language. Their study is in some ways comparable to that described earlier by Halle, Marshall and Spradlin (1979). As in the study by Ivancic *et al.* (1981), part of the thinking was that teaching could advantageously be undertaken in the context of daily care activities.

Some of the same residents with profound retardation and the two with hearing impairment were involved, and hence began this phase of the intervention with some knowledge of nine signs, a number increased here to 17. The teaching was carried out in the residents' living units. The procedure employed modified incidental teaching with provision made for staff frequently to prompt signing by the students rather than simply waiting for them to sign so that they could reinforce the behaviour. Three strategies were used. First, the physical environment was changed to include a 'reinforcer display' — a shelf or table — on which objects of value to the residents were placed. If a student signed that he or she wanted one of these objects it was given along with praise. If no sign was given in the first five seconds, the staff member asked one or more questions about what the student wanted, or about the object in order to elicit the sign. Again, reinforcement followed correct production of the sign. Failure to produce the sign led to manual guidance by the staff member. If residents did not approach the objects, then they were gently guided to the table or shelf. Second, routine staff-resident interactions were altered in such a way that during ordinary interactions staff incorporated signing into the interaction and prompted residents. Third, short training sessions were introduced intermittently during the day, single items being signed and discussed.

In contrast to the first intervention, this procedure led to spontaneous signing by residents in their living units. Staff reported that the intervention had not interfered with their carrying out routine activities. Though Total Communication was employed, increase in vocalisation was not observed with any consistency across students. This study demonstrates well the desirability of carrying communication teaching, whether spoken or signed, into the actual environment and ensuring that the student is motivated to use what has been learnt to influence that environment.

Similar concerns regarding the validity of the signs learnt for the students informed Wilson's (1983) incorporation of a manual signing programme into a classroom for children who were profoundly retarded and deaf-blind. Five such children with these characteristics were selected from the class for this Australian programme. The CA of these children was around 7 years at the start of the intervention, with their mean level of cognition at 5 months, receptive and expressive language at 4 and 3 months respectively. Their daily living development, however, was appreciably higher, 16–27 months in different areas. Given the sensorimotor abilities required to achieve these levels in self-help, this might be a more realistic reflection of their cognitive achievement, the five month assessment being a gross under-estimate. Certainly the assumption that they were cognitively at or beyond Stage VI sensorimotor development would be consistent with the studies of Kahn and others and would leave them on the border of profound-severe mental retardation. The five children had bilateral hearing losses ranging from severe (75–90dB) to profound (90dB+). It was not possible to assess visual acuity, but four of the children were classified as severely visually impaired and responded only to intense visual stimuli, while the fifth was completely blind. All showed bizarre behaviour (e.g. head banging, eye poking, etc.).

A repertoire of signs was selected by those who knew the children's needs and environment. The system chosen was the Australian Sign Language with English word order followed and Total Communication being employed. The programme consisted of three phases: I: Receptive skills. II: Signing of nouns represented in objects and pictures. III: Verb-noun combination with generalisation to novel combinations. Staff working in the classroom with the children undertook the teaching.

In phase 1 the teacher signed a concept clearly in front of the child, speaking the word(s) at the same time. Much of this teaching took place at snack times and 'pour juice' would be an example signed to the child. The sign was considered learnt when the child responded appropriately to it on five consecutive occasions.

In phase II the children themselves were taught to sign using the following means:

(i) *Moulding*: Applicable to concrete objects which are put in the child's hands and the sign is moulded by the teacher — a technique particularly appropriate to the blind or partially sighted child.

(ii) *Shaping:* Here an actual object is not employed and hence signs for abstract concepts can be taught.

(iii) *Imitation:* Employed in the tactile mode in cases where visual impairment precludes visual observation of the model.

Wilson describes the basic strategy (pp. 161–2) which entails imitation, physical prompting and reinforcement.

In phase III, noun-verb combinations and their generalisation were taught. In similar fashion to some of the programmes involving spoken noun-verb combinations, the child has to learn to follow instructions such as 'point to book' or 'give chair'.

Entry into the programme took the longest time, i.e. getting underway in phase 1. Nevertheless, after 18 months all the children responded to their own name signs and to several one- and two-sign instructions. In phase II, after six months, the children each made up a minimum of 18 signs, one of them achieving 33 signs. These signs were for common objects and abstract nouns such as colour. A learning-to-learn effect was also noted with an increasingly rapid acquisition of new signs. In phase III, after six months, the children had learnt 36 noun-verb combinations and were able to generalise to novel combinations. Assessment of parallel areas of development during the course of the programme when compared to the development of children in a contrast group not taught signing led to two further conclusions drawn by Wilson:

The positive changes that can be brought about when the ability to communicate is increased include a decrease in self-stimulatory, destructive, and self-abusive behaviours. The most noteworthy fact about the children's progress in developing communication skills is that the gains in communication have been accompanied by gains in social interaction and concept formation; also the achievements of the communication programme have proved beneficial to both the self-help skills programme and the perception programme. (p. 167)

She goes on:

Their horizons have widened as they have come into contact with people who want to communicate with them, and they have found they can respond. All children in the demonstration group are now signing in a variety of different settings and with a variety of people, not just the staff involved in the classroom. (p. 169).

Using Aided Devices

McDonald (1976) has described the general strategy that should be pursued in introducing a communication board. At the outset it is necessary to establish that the person can match an object to its representation in picture form, and that attention and memory abilities are adequate to the task. In addition, the person must be able to point reliably. Physical consideration must be taken into account when the individual is not ambulant, as is likely to be the case. Adequate support should be given to maintain general posture and head control. Though the demands of physical therapy may dictate that such supports are not desirable throughout the day, some balance must be achieved between physical and communicative development. Similarly, adequate visual assessment must be undertaken to ensure that the objects illustrated can be seen (see Chapter 1 of this volume). The content of the items on the board should be individualised and significant people in the person's life should aid in the selection. Where necessary, alternative modes to manual pointing should be devised, e.g. head pointing, direction of gaze, etc.

Reid and Hurblut (1977) report a study which in most respects amply illustrates the approach advocated by McDonald and which is highly relevant to the group with whom we are concerned. While no specific IQs are reported, it is suggested that all were below IQ = 36 and major physical impairments were clearly present. Four people participated in the study:

> *Jill:* a 34 year old female with a medical diagnosis of spastic paralysis with generalized athetosis and encephalopathy due to injury at birth. She was restricted to sitting or a horizontal position due to skeletal deformities.
> *Pete:* a 34 year old with medical diagnosis including encephalopathy, *grand mal* seizure activity, and spastic paralysis generalized with athetosis. He was confined to a horizontal position.
> *Robert:* a 31 year old male described in his medical file as being severely retarded physically and as very spastic. Robert was restricted to a semi-horizontal position with seriously contracted legs.
> *Victor:* a 33 year old male with severe spasticity. He was restricted to a horizontal position due to severe muscle rigidity. (pp. 392–3)

Staff who had worked for some time with these residents could communicate with them, successfully employing idiosyncratic cues such as eye movements and small movements of their limbs. With unfamiliar people, however, communication was not possible. Reid and Hurblut (1977) adopted a three-stage strategy that reflects many of the elements of McDonald's approach. Teaching first was aimed at establishing co-ordinated movement that would permit pointing to the communication board. Second, pointing to pictures of significance to the residents was taught. Finally, generalisation of the learned communication was determined.

The nature of the pointing was adapted to the four individuals. In the cases of Jill, Pete and Victor a device was attached to their heads with a pointer on it that could be seen by them if they brought it into contact with the picture and word on the communication board. This was established in conjunction with a physiotherapist who determined degree of head control and range of movement, an input that emphasises the need for interdisciplinary collaboration in this area of aided communication. Robert was able to use his hand.

For all four residents, co-ordination was taught by the teacher indicating a block on the communication board and asking the student to 'Point to the block'. This was taught using verbal instructions, praise, corrective feedback and manual guidance with repeated practice in pointing. Correct pointing was reinforced by using praise. Though co-ordination never achieved perfection, it increased reliably and sufficiently to move into the communication phase.

Communication was concerned with leisure activities with a view to making the programme a first step in developing leisure-related skills. Five areas of the building related to leisure were illustrated on pictures with the appropriate word written underneath, e.g. television room, radio room and so on. Initially the students learnt to identify the areas by pointing on instruction, e.g. 'Show me where you would point if you wanted to go to the television room'. A similar procedure was used as in the co-ordination training though manual guidance was not employed. Generalisation was established by asking for an indication of the correct picture in the actual leisure area, i.e. 'Show me where you are'. Victor was excluded from this phase as he was able at the outset to indicate the areas. The other three, however, learnt to indicate the correct picture in response to the pointing request. Generalisation was demonstrated, though imperfectly.

In the final, social validation phase, a comparison was made between the success in communication by the residents with and without the communication board with strangers. None was able correctly to interpret what was being communicated without the board. With it, however, communication was 100 per cent successful.

A careful consideration of this study will show that it meets many of the requirements of ecological intervention we have noted. The content of the communications were highly relevant to the person's life and indeed much of the training and evaluation took place in real-life settings. The adaptive value of the procedure was shown by generalisation to people who would have failed entirely to understand the communicative attempts of the resident.

A move from pictures towards more symbolic material would increase the flexibility of communication, however, and for some individuals with profound retardation and multiple impairments such an extension is feasible. We have already summarised Welch and Pear's (1980) programme which successfully taught Cathy, a child with profound retardation and cerebral palsy, to use Blissymbols on a communication board. Harris-Vanderheiden (1977) reports a more extended application of such teaching with a group of physically impaired children of varying degrees of intellectual retardation. The five who participated lived in a large institution and were selected on the basis of criteria several of which are the same as those noted by Shane: (i) object permanence achieved; (ii) ability to establish eye contact; (iii) ability to attend to task for five minutes; (iv) physically impaired to such a degree that manual signing and finger spelling are precluded; (v) picture and word boards had been tried and failed.

A Total Communication approach was employed in which the teacher spoke when the child started to select the appropriate symbol. The programme began with the Blissymbols for 'Yes' and 'No' responses which in some idiosyncratic way the children could already indicate. It then progressed to 'eat' and 'drink' and the use of symbols to answer questions. As the child became more competent, so the symbols were posted on the appropriate objects in the child's environment. The programme was initiated during its first few months by specialists in teaching communication but was then maintained by care staff with an evaluation after 16 months. For child 'A', an 11 year old who was quadriplegic and microcephalic, 100 symbols of 2–4 unit length were being used in comprehension and expression after 16 months. At the same follow-up, child 'B' who had cerebral palsy was employing 25 symbols in comprehension in 1–2 unit length. Child 'C', 14 years, and described as cerebral palsied and severely mentally retarded, had acquired 125 symbols (2–4 unit length) and was using these expressively and comprehensively. Child 'D', 12 years, cerebral palsied, moved from use of symbols and into reading and a sight word vocabulary and was finally regarded as only educable retarded. Child 'E' was 11 years and is described as mentally retarded acquired 200 symbols employing them expressively and comprehensively. In relation to the children whom we would regard as profoundly retarded and multiply impaired, the authors note that 7–30 symbols could be learnt and used comprehensively.

Both the reports we have summarised were concerned with retardation and physical impairment. Jackson (1984) describes the extension of Blissymbols to multiply impaired children with visual impairments. This is achieved through use of the *Cheyne Symbol System* — 'Tactile Bliss'. The system was devised at the Cheyne Walk Spastic Centre in London and attempts to provide a simple form of expression coded by means of tactile picto- and ideographic symbols derived from Blissymbolics but differentiated in texture. Three distinctions are used: (i) engraving; (ii) raising, e.g. with wire stuck on the card; (iii) difference in surface texture, e.g. sandpaper on smooth background. These are arranged on a communication board and a vocabulary of 112 items is available. We have not come across any published studies evaluating this development of Blissymbolics for people with profound retardation and multiple impairments. In an unpublished note, Lovelace (undated) describes the use of tactile Bliss with a six and a half year old child with Joubert's Syndrome who was nonambulant, severely visually impaired and self-mutilating. Lack of functional vision precluded successful use of manual signing though BSL-M had been attempted. Again, a communication board approach was adopted and in the early stages of the programme he was able to select five symbols differentiated in terms of materials of varying textures.

References

Ausman, J.A. and Gaddy, M.R. (1974) 'Reinforcement Training for Echolalia: Developing a Repertoire of Appropriate Responses in an Echolalic Girl', *Mental Retardation, 12,* 20–1

Barton, E.S. (1970) 'Operant Conditioning of Appropriate and Inappropriate Social Speech in the Profoundly Retarded', *Journal of Mental Deficiency Research, 17,* 183–91

Bricker, D., Dennison, L. and Bricker, W. (1976) *A Language Intervention Program for Developmentally Young Children,* Mailman Center for Child Development Monograph 1, Miami

Coupe, J., Barton, L., Barber, M., Collins, L., Levy, D. and Murphy, D. (1985) *An Introduction to the Affective Communication Assessment,* Manchester Education Committee, Manchester

DeHaven, E.D. and Garcia, E.E. (1974) 'Continuation of Training as a Variable Influencing the Generalization of Speech in a Retarded Child', *Journal of Abnormal Child Psychology, 2,* 217–27

Duker, P.C. and Morsink, H. (1984) 'Acquisiton and Cross-Setting Generalisation of Manual Signs with Retarded Individuals', *Journal of Applied Behavior Analysis, 17,* 93–103

Faw, G.D., Reid, D.H., Schepis, M.M., Fitzgerald, J.R. and Welty, P.A. (1981) 'Involving Institutional Staff in the Development and Maintenance of Sign

Language Skills with Profoundly Retarded Persons', *Journal of Applied Behavior Analysis, 14,* 411–23

Ferrier, L.J. and Shane, H.C. (1983) 'A Description of a Non-speaking Population under Consideration for Augmentative Communication Systems' in J. Hogg and P.J. Mittler (eds.), *Advances in Mental Handicap Research: Volume 2: Aspects of Competence in Mentally Handicapped People,* Wiley, Chichester

Fraser, W.I. and Ozols, D. (1981) 'He Sounds and Looks Sore — Professionals' Evaluations of the Profoundly Handicapped Person's Pain and Distress Signals' in W.I. Fraser and R. Grieve (eds.), *Communicating with Normal and Retarded Children,* Wright and Son, Bristol

Fristoe, M. and Lloyd, L.L. (1978) 'A Survey of the Use of Non-speech Systems with the Severely Communication Impaired', *Mental Retardation, 16,* 99–103

Garcia, E.E. (1974) 'The Training and Generalization of a Conversational Speech Form in Nonverbal Retardates, *Journal of Applied Behavior Analysis, 7,* 137–9

Garcia, E.E. and DeHaven, E.D. (1980) 'Teaching Generalized Speech: Re-establishing a Previously Trained Repertoire of Functional Speech', *Behavior Research of Severe Developmental Disabilities, 1,* 147–60

Goodman, L., Wilson, P.S. and Bornstein, H. (1978) 'Results of a National Survey of Sign Language Programmes in Special Education', *Mental Retardation, 16,* 104–6

Guess, D., Sailor, W. and Baer, D.M. (1978) *Functional Speech and Language Training for the Severely Handicapped,* H. & H. Enterprises, Lawrence, Ks.

Guess, D., Sailor, W., Keogh, W.J. and Baer, D.M. (1976) 'Language Development Programs for Severely Handicapped Children' in N. Haring and L. Brown (eds.), *Teaching the Severely Handicapped: Vol. 1,* Grune and Stratton, New York

Halle, J.W., Marshall, A.M. and Spradlin, J.E. (1979) 'Time Delay: A Technique to Increase Language Use and Facilitate Generalization in Retarded Children', *Journal of Applied Behavior Analysis, 12,* 431–9

Harris, S.L. (1975) 'Teaching Language to Nonverbal Children — With an Emphasis on Problems of Generalization', *Psychological Bulletin, 85,* 565–80

Harris-Vanderheiden, D. (1977) 'Blissymbols and the Mentally Retarded' in C.G. Vanderheiden and K. Grilley (eds.), *Non-vocal Communication Techniques and Aids for the Severely Physically Handicapped,* University Park Press, Baltimore

Ivancic, M.T., Reid, D.H., Iwata, B.A., Faw, G.D. and Page, T.J. (1981) 'Evaluating a Supervision Program for Developing and Maintaining Therapeutic Staff-Resident Interactions During Institutional Care Routines', *Journal of Applied Behavior Analysis, 14,* 95–107

Jackson, M. (1984) 'The Cheyne Symbol System: A New Approach to Language through Touch for the Multi-handicapped Blind Child', *British Journal of Visual Impairment, 11,* 12–16

Jones, L.M., Reid, B.D. and Kiernan, C.C. (1982) 'Signs and Symbols: The 1980 Survey' in M. Peter and R. Barnes (eds.), *Signs, Symbols and Schools,* NCSE, Stratford

Kahn, J.V. (1975) 'Relationship of Piaget's Sensorimotor Period to Language Acquisition of Profoundly Retarded Children', *American Journal of Mental Deficiency, 79,* 640–3

Kahn, J.V. (1984) 'Cognitive Training and Initial Use of Referential Speech',

Topics in Language Disorders, December, 14–28

Kiernan, C.C. (1983) 'The Exploration of Sign and Symbol Effects' in J. Hogg and P.J. Mittler (eds.), *Advances in Mental Handicap Research: Vol. 2: Aspects of Competence in Mentally Handicapped People,* Wiley, Chichester

Kiernan, C.C. (1984) 'Nonspeech Communication in the UK: Editorial', *Journal of Mental Deficiency Research, 28,* 1–2

Kiernan, C.C. (1985) 'Communication' in A.M. Clarke, A.D.B. Clarke and J.M. Berg (eds.), *Mental Deficiency: The Changing Outlook,* 4th edn, Methuen, London

Kiernan, C.C., Reid, B.D. and Jones, L.M. (1982) *Signs and Symbols: A Review of Literature and Survey of Use on Non-vocal Communication Systems,* University of London Institute of Education, London

Kohl, F., Fundakowski, G., Menchetti, B. and Coleman, S. (1977) 'Manual Communication Training for Severely Handicapped Students' in J.M. Cronin (ed.), *The Severely and Handicapped Child: Proceedings from the 1977 Statewide Institute for Educators of the Severely and Profoundly Handicapped,* Specialized Educational Services, Illinois

Lavatelli, C.S. (1970a) *Early Childhood Curriculum: A Piagetian Program,* American Science and Engineering Company, Boston

Lavatelli, C.S. (1970b) *Teacher's Guide to Accompanying Early Childhood Curriculum and to Supplement Piaget's Theory Applied to an Early Childhood Curriculum,* American Science and Engineering Company, Boston

Light, P., Remington, R. and Porter, D. (1982) 'Substitutes for Speech: Nonvocal Approaches to Communication' in M. Beveridge (ed.), *Children's Thinking Through Language,* Edward Arnold, London

Lloyd, L.L. and Karlan, G.R. (1984) 'Current Topics: Non-speech Communication Symbols and Systems: Where have we been and where are we going?', *Journal of Mental Deficiency Research, 28,* 3–20

Lovelace, P. (undated) 'Experimenting with a Tactile Form of Blissymbols for a Profoundly Visually Impaired Young Child, with Learning Difficulties', unpublished manuscript

McCuller, W.R. and Salzberg, C.L. (1984) 'Generalized Action-object Verbal Instruction-following by Profoundly Mentally Retarded Adults', *American Journal of Mental Deficiency, 88,* 442–5

McDonald, E.T. (1976) 'Design and Application of Communication Boards' in C.G. Vanderheiden and K. Grilley (eds.), *Non-vocal Communication Techniques and Aids for the Severely Physically Handicapped,* University Park Press, Baltimore

McLean, J. and Synder-McLean, L.K. (1984) 'Recent Developments in Pragmatics: Remedial Implications' in D.J. Muller (ed.), *Remediating Children's Language: Behavioural and Naturalistic Approaches,* Croom Helm, London/College-Hill Press, San Diego

McLean, J. and Snyder-Mclean, L.K. (1985) 'Developmentally Early Communicative Behaviors Among Severely Mentally Retarded Adolescents', Seminar Topic Outline, Hester Adrian Research Centre, University of Manchester, Manchester

Miller, J.F. and Yoder, D.E. (1972) 'A Syntax Teaching Program' in J.E. McLean, D. Yoder and R.L. Schiefelbusch (eds.), *Language Intervention with the Retarded,* University Park Press, Baltimore

Miller, J.F. and Yoder, D.E. (1974) 'An Ontogenetic Language Teaching Strategy for Retarded Children' in R.L. Schiefelbusch and L.L. Lloyd (eds.), *Language Perspectives: Acquisition, Retardation and Intervention*, Pro-Ed, Inc. Austin, Tex.

Reid, D.H. and Hurblut, B. (1977) 'Teaching Nonvocal Communication Skills to Multihandicapped Retarded Adults', *Journal of Applied Behavior Analysis*, *10*, 591–603

Remington, R. and Light, P. (1983) 'Some Problems in the Evaluation of Research on Non-oral Communication Systems', in J. Hogg and P.J. Mittler (eds.), *Advances in Mental Handicap Research: Volume 2: Aspects of Competence in Mentally Handicapped People*, Wiley, Chichester

Rogers-Warren, A.K., Warren, S.F. and Baer, D.M. (1983) 'Interactional Basis of Language Learning' in K.T. Kernan, M.J. Begab and R.B. Edgerton (eds.), *Environments and Behavior: The Adaptation of Mentally Retarded Persons*, University Park Press, Baltimore

Schepis, M.M., Reid, D.H., Fitzgerald, J.R., Faw, G.D., van den Pol, R.A. and Welty, P.A. (1982) 'A Program for Increasing Manual Signing by Autistic and Profoundly Retarded Youth within the Daily Environment', *Journal of Applied Behavior Analysis, 15*, 363–79

Schreibman, L.C. and Carr, E.G. (1978) 'Elimination of Echolalic Responses to Questions through the Training of a Generalized Verbal Response', *Journal of Applied Behavior Analysis, 11*, 453–63

Shane, H.C. (1981) 'Decision Making in Early Augmentative Communication System Use' in R.L. Schiefelbusch and D.D. Bricker (eds.), *Early Language: Acquisition and Intervention*, University Park Press, Baltimore

Shane, H.C. and Bashir, A.S. (1980) 'Election Criteria for Determining Candidacy for an Augmentative Communication System: Preliminary Considerations', *Journal of Speech and Hearing Disorders, 45*, 408–14

Sternberg, L., McNerney, C.D. and Pegnatore, L. (1985) 'Developing Co-Active Imitative Behaviors with Profoundly Mentally Handicapped Students', *Education and Training of the Mentally Retarded, 20*, 260–7

Sternberg, L. and Owens, A. (1985) 'Establishing Pre-language Signaling Behavior with Profoundly Mentally Handicapped Students: A Preliminary Investigation', *Journal of Mental Deficiency Research, 28*, 81–93

Sternberg, L. Pegnatore, L. and Hill, C. (1983) 'Establishing Interactive Communication Behaviors with Profoundly Mentally Handicapped Students', *Journal of the Association of the Severely Handicapped, 8*, 39–46

Tawney, J. and Hipsher, L. (1972) 'Systematic Instruction for Retarded Children: The Illinois Program (Part II): Systematic Language Instruction', State of Illinois, Office of the Superintendent of Public Instruction

VanBiervliet, A., Spangler, P. and Marshall, A.M. (1979) 'An Ecological Approach for Increasing Language During Mealtimes', Paper presented to the Association for Behavior Analysis', June, Dearborn, Michigan

Vanderheiden, G.C. (1976) 'Providing the Child with a Means to Indicate' in G.C. Vanderheiden and K. Grilley (eds.), *Non-vocal Communication Techniques and Aids for the Severely Physically Handicapped*, University Park Press, Baltimore

Vanderheiden, G.C. and Grilley, K. (eds.) (1976) *Non-vocal Communication Techniques and Aids for the Severely Physically Handicapped*, University

Park Press, Baltimore

Warner, J. (1981a) *Helping the Handicapped Child with Early Feeding: A Manual for Parents and Professionals*, Winslow Press, Buckingham

Warner, J. (1981b) 'Teaching the Profoundly Handicapped Child: Feeding and the Development of Early Speech Sounds', unpublished manuscript, University of Manchester

Warren, S.F. and Rogers-Warren, A.K. (1983) 'Because No One Asked . . . Affecting the Generalization of Trained Vocabulary within a Residential Institution' in K.T. Kernan, M.J. Begab and R.B. Edgerton (eds.), *Environments and Behavior: The Adaptation of Mentally Retarded Persons*, University Park Press, Baltimore

Welch, S.J. and Pears, J.J. (1980) 'Generalisation of Naming Responses to Objects in the Natural Environment as a Function of Training Stimulus Modality with Retarded Children', *Journal of Applied Behavior Analysis*, *13*, 629–43

Wilson, A.R.S. (1983) 'The Use of Manual Communication with Deaf-Blind Mentally Handicapped Children' in J. Hogg and P.J. Mittler (eds.), *Advances in Mental Handicap Research: Volume 2: Aspects of Competence in Mentally Handicapped People*, Wiley, Chichester

5 INTERVENTION IN MOTOR DEVELOPMENT AND COMPETENCE

Introduction

All behaviour is dependent for its realisation on motor activity, whether the behaviour is spoken or signed language or those activities we have called 'cognitive'. Damage to, or abnormality of, the central nervous system (CNS) resulting in shortcomings in motor activity has wide-ranging consequences for the individual's ability to adapt to the environment and intervention to improve this situation is central to remediation. We have already seen that individuals with profound retardation have a high probability of physical impairments arising from CNS damage (Volume 1, Chapter 1) and any curriculum for this group will entail a major effort to improve or circumvent such impairments.

At the outset we need to distinguish between three aspects of motor impairment. First, motor dysfunction can arise from damage to the CNS and be reflected in one or more of the cerebral palsies or other forms of motor dysfunction such as spina bifida. Secondly, motor development can be slow, with the typical milestones related to postural control, body mobility and hand function being achieved appreciably later than for nonhandicapped children. Thirdly, the achievement of competent motor behaviour, notably in upper limb use, can be delayed or ineffective through cognitive shortcomings. Motor competence of this sort, of course, is typically tapped in early nursery tasks such as formboards as well as in self-help abilities such as spoon use.

Motor dysfunction, delayed development and incompetence are in reality intertwined. Any form of dysfunction will almost certainly slow development and make competent performance of a variety of tasks difficult if not impossible. In addition, the strong cognitive component underlying motor competence will be a powerful influence on such ability. In working with people who are profoundly retarded we are all familiar with the individual who has the motor ability to retrieve a hidden object, but whose understanding of the permanence of objects precludes reaching and taking the object. For the purpose of formulating an intervention strategy, however, the distinction between dysfunction, development and competence needs to be borne in mind. Not only does it have implication for the nature of programming, but also for the relative inputs of the interdisciplinary team and the relation between their activities. Both physiotherapist and teacher have crucial contributions to make in the area of motor intervention, though we can define a shift in their relative inputs as we move from dysfunction, through development to motor competence.

The emphasis in this chapter is on the context and background of motor intervention rather than on the details of different approaches. There is an extensive literature on therapeutic aspects of such intervention with which those working with people with profound retardation and multiple impairments should be familiar. These range from short, well-illustrated pamphlets to extensive but accessible handbooks. A number will be cited and described. Similarly, the many, often conflicting, theoretical positions that underlie therapy need to be commented on, however briefly. In this chapter, then, we attempt to provide an overview that covers the main issues and points the reader to specific examples of both general programmes and those concerned with a given piece of motor behaviour. We begin with a discussion on assessment then move on to an account of the overall context in which intervention should be carried out. This is followed by a consideration of intervention and motor dysfunction which begins with a description of some of the more frequently employed techniques and their theoretical background: we then describe some specific studies. Finally, motor programming in the sense of improving motor competence is discussed.

Assessment

Professionals working with people with developmental retardation have drawn extensively on the many developmental checklists that chart change in postural control, body mobility and hand function. The Motor Scale of the Bayley Scales of Development (Bayley 1969) or the Gross Motor Scale of the Griffith's Mental Development Scales (Griffiths 1970) represent familiar instruments devised respectively in the USA and the UK. It is essentially modified versions of such scales that have typically been employed to monitor intervention with people with developmental delay. Thus, the Gross Motor Skill Scale of the Portage system (Shearer and Shearer 1972) and the Anson House Gross and Fine Motor Checklists (Gunstone 1979, revised 1985) present developments deriving from the standardised scales. The value of such instruments and the many others that have been developed in schools, adult centres and other settings, is that they provide a broad framework of normative development against which to view the motor status of individuals with profound impairments. Several limitations should also be noted, however:

(i)   Such checklists provide a starting point for intervention, i.e. they 'place' the person somewhere between developmental milestones. They are too coarse-grained to provide monitoring instruments for individuals whose rate of progress is extremely slow nor do they provide information on the relation of a given milestone to other prerequisites that are essential to the emergence of that behaviour.

(ii) By their very nature, standardised scales do not permit environmental adaptations in order to allow the person to show the behaviour of interest. Thus, no provision is made for assessing mobility in relation to a given orthopaedic intervention.

(iii) While a starting point for intervention may be indicated by such scales, they have not been conceived in a framework that relates to the chosen therapeutic approach.

The first two of the above criticisms of developmental checklists can be dealt with by what Mira (1977) and Guess, Rues, Warren, Lyon, Mulligan, Lehr, Janssen, Murphy, Fosage and Barnes (1979) refer to as a shift from such qualitative assessment to quantitative. Here specific defined behaviours are monitored with respect to their duration and frequency in a way which permits fine-grain analysis and monitoring of change. This is essentially an applied analysis of behaviour strategy and Guess *et al.* (1979) summarise what is entailed:

(i)   The behaviour must be clearly defined in such a way that independent observers can agree upon its occurrence. For example 'head erect' might, they suggest, be defined as 'the head is considered to be in an erect position when no part of the head or neck (chin to clavicle) is touching the child's arms which are in contact with the supporting surface' (p. 23).

(ii) The conditions of observation are exactly specified with respect to positioning and handling of the person, setting, and possibly time of day.

(iii) The equipment and apparatus to be employed are specified.

In addition, some statement regarding the conditions under which generalisation will be displayed if called for.

Mira (1977) suggests that by employing such an approach, detailed monitoring of progress is possible of behaviours that are clinically and functionally relevant to the person. The importance of such a strategy is clearly shown by a study of children with profound retardation and multiple impairments by Sebba (1978). Here behavioural programmes were quantitatively monitored as advocated by Mira and by Guess *et al.* and Motor Scores on the Bayley Psychomotor Scale assessed. Despite demonstrable progress on individual programmes, these were not detected on relevant Bayley Scale items. Thus, child 'SA' showed improvement on both grasping and arm raising but only limited change in psychomotor age (PMA) over the period the programmes were in operation. 'HJ' showed improvement in sitting up from supine but regression to her original PMA following a slight increase during the intervention. Sebba concludes that the comparison of the Bayley scores and the individual programme-related developments suggests that changes in the quality or quantity of specific behaviours monitored by the programmes are not reflected in scores on test. The Bayley items appear to advance in larger steps than those made on specific programmes and subtle differences are not noted on the test.

The third point above can be overcome by assessment that is functional, i.e. is undertaken in such a way that its function with respect to the intended future therapy is known. Both total and specific therapies are carried out to plan the programme, as suggested by Levitt (1982), who goes on to emphasise that simply listing motor function is not enough. Assessment for both therapy and daily care permits: (i) Planning of programmes. (ii) Assessment of progress. (iii) The addition of further observations to the picture already built up. Levitt (1982) goes on to emphasise the need to assess the person in the parallel developmental channels of prone, supine, sitting, standing and walking development. An illustrative chart showing the major phases of development in these areas is given (Levitt 1982 pp. 240–1). In addition, hand function is also assessed. While Levitt's approach is directed to cerebral palsy, though readily extendable to other forms of motor dysfunction, Holle (1976) deals with motor retardation generally. Her book also contains a separate wall chart covering motor development to 6 years of age. Levitt, too, discusses assessment of abnormal motor performance (as distinct from developmental assessment) and of deformity (pp. 51–62).

The approach to assessment is also critical to collecting valid information. Levitt notes that the following strategy should be followed:

(i)   Observation of spontaneous motor behaviour in natural settings.

(ii)   Where children are concerned, the therapist should establish rapport with the parent in the child's presence.

(iii)   Avoidance of a formal test or examination atmosphere.

(iv)   Time should be taken and no impression of hurry given.

(v)   Child should only be undressed when this is acceptable to him or her.

(vi)   The order in which the information is gathered is irrelevant, there being no need to follow a prescribed sequence.

(vii)   Observation and assessment continues through therapy.

(viii) Early attempts at therapy during the preliminary phases of therapy can provide valuable exploratory information.

(ix)   Several sessions may be needed.

(x)   Treatment can facilitate behaviours not observed during assessment of spontaneous motor behaviour.

Where the individual being assessed can in some way be instructed in executing a given action, consideration needs to be given as to how best this can be achieved. Modelling an action is a favoured method, though a recent study by Tomporowski and Ellis (1984) casts doubt on this. Working with ambulant adults, some of whom were profoundly retarded, they compared modelling of gross motor actions and graduated guidance. Modelling involved demonstration of the required behaviour and verbalising what the response was. Graduated guidance began with a verbal prompt, followed by a verbal and gestural prompt such as pointing. Physical guidance was then employed using the minimum amount of force necessary, i.e. the person was put through the movement. Verbal praise and physical contact followed successful performance of the action in both cases. While physical guidance was more effective than modelling with individuals who were severely retarded, both techniques failed with those who were profoundly retarded. The authors suggest that extensive training might be necessary for preparing such individuals for motor assessment.

The qualitative and quantitative approaches to assessment outlined above are not only complementary but in several respects have features in common. Both entail rigorous observations in the early phases and are continued while the intervention is in progress. Both are undertaken in relation to improvement in adaptive functioning and proponents of both positions emphasise that the ultimate criterion of much motor programming is the improvement of performance in everyday tasks and situations.

The Context for Intervention

We have already noted that there is a continuum of assessment from that involving specialist evaluations by a physiotherapist through to more obviously curriculum-oriented activities for which a teacher or trainer may have undertaken observations. This continuum is also involved when we come to implementing programmes. Levitt emphasises that the motor assessments she describes lead to programmes that should be executed or supervised by the physiotherapist:

> These should be carried out by qualified physiotherapists and occupational therapists and shown to anyone caring for the motor-delayed and disabled child. Where techniques require a physiotherapist only, they are labelled 'physiotherapy suggestions'. Techniques taught to others are labelled 'treatment suggestions and daily care'. Selection of the appropriate technique for each child should be made by therapists and when necessary discussed with doctors and other team members. (p. 68)

Such discussion is clearly a two-way process. The teacher or trainer involved will have more extensive experience of the person's behaviour in everyday life situations and a fuller understanding of both the motivational characteristics and the intellectual abilities of the client. In line with Levitt's emphasis on taking the whole person into account in formulating a programme, weight must be given within the interdisciplinary team to this input.

Levitt's suggestion that some recommendations by the physiotherapists can be implemented by other team members is of crucial importance when in most situations the time available to physiotherapists to undertake therapy is woefully inadequate. While there is no substitute for direct involvement by a physiotherapist in this process, useful illustrated booklets do exist for teachers and trainers to brief themselves on physical therapy. Hollis (1977a) emphasises that her own booklet is not intended to provide a 'do-it-yourself' physiotherapy book. This publication and the accompanying booklet (Hollis 1977b) both provide valuable guidance on the basic areas of motor development noted above with the exception of hand function. In far greater detail and richly illustrated is Finnie's (1974) book *Handling the Young Cerebral Palsied Child at Home* which should be required reading for anyone having to lift, move and position physically impaired children of the kind with which this book is concerned.

All recent accounts of physical therapy with people with retardation and additional impairments distinguish between the specialised input of the physiotherapist who should exclusively carry out certain interventions, and his or her role in transmitting those skills to other professionals and parents concerned with the individual. With respect to the latter Levitt (1982) emphasises that *selection* of techniques for use by others is the physiotherapist's responsibility. Almond (1982) describes this inter-disciplinary role of the physiotherapist in the setting of a preschool group of nonhandicapped and handicapped children some of whom were both profoundly retarded and physically impaired.

From these opening concerns with assessment and setting we now move to a consideration of the theoretical background of intervention.

Intervention and Motor Dysfunction

In this section we describe a little of the theoretical background to intervention aimed at remediating motor dysfunction and its consequences and some of the basic techniques employed. Our intention is not to be in any way comprehensive at either the level of theory or practice. It is simply to give teachers and trainers some awareness of the main ideas and concepts involved in order to permit them to understand more fully the approach of physiotherapists and the relevance of their expertise to the clients.

Some Theoretical Positions

All professionals and many parents concerned with people whose disabilities result from brain damage will have encountered a variety of named therapies each of which has its proponents. Here we briefly describe those that we have encountered most frequently in relation to people who are multiply impaired and profoundly retarded. Where specific information exists on the effectiveness of a given procedure with this population we shall also consider the relevant findings. While some of these approaches are concerned centrally with motor function, others deal with this aspect within a much wider framework as is the case with co-active therapy with which we begin. It should also be added that other positions are used to inform intervention with the wider population of motor-impaired children and brief summaries will be found in Levitt (1982 pp. 24–32).

Co-active Therapy. A fuller description of co-active therapy has been given in Chapter 2, pp. 83–5. With respect to multiply impaired people McInnes and Treffry (1982) describe the use of the approach with gross motor behaviour (pp. 94ff.) and fine motor behaviour (p. 141). The theoretical basis for the approach rests in the work of Van Dijk (1977) who emphasises the motor basis of cognition and the importance of anticipation by the person of motor movement patterns as a means of establishing contact with external reality. As noted, the technique is directed to deaf-blind individuals of differing ability levels and with respect to gross motor behaviour the actual skills noted range beyond likely activites for people with profound retardation and multiple impairments. Nevertheless, a detailed curriculum is offered (pp. 100–40) that embraces the application of co-active techniques to children who are multiply impaired and at low levels of intellectual functioning. Thus, critical areas such as head control, body awareness, rolling, balance, sitting, crawling, standing, raising to standing and walking begin the sequence and roller and ice skating and swimming complete it. With respect to head control, for example, the methods and activities advocated are as follows:

(i)   General co-operation between child and therapist must first be established.
(ii) Next, manipulation through the activity is undertaken.
(iii) A variety of different stimuli — tactile, auditory and visual — are employed to increase curiosity.
(iv) The communicative sequence advocated throughout the approach is employed.

Similarly, fine motor activities range from reflex grasp of an object placed in the hand, through basic sensorimotor schemes such as hand-to-mouth and sucking, play with hands in mid-line, transfer of objects from hand to hand through to screwing lids on jars and use of scissors. Methods and activities are described.

Conductive Education. As described in Chapter 2, co-active therapy is effectively a comprehensive educational system directed primarily at enhancing motor development and competence rather than dealing with dysfunction in its own right. Conductive therapy can also be described in such broad educational terms, but the starting point for the technique was not sensory impairment but specific physical impairment. The technique originated from Andras Peto who founded the State Institute for the Motor Disabled in Budapest for the treatment of cerebral palsy, dystrophies, paraplegias and spina bifida. The background to the Institute and the approach are described by Cotton (1965), Cotton and Parnwell (1968) and Cottam and Sutton (1985). Cotton and Parnwell (1968) describe the basis of conductive education as requiring that 'all the different aspects of education, whether physical, mental or therapeutic, are so integrated under conditions deliberately suited to the child's brain damaged condition as to make it possible for him to learn' (p. 50).

This need for integration leads to a single individual in charge of all aspects of the child's education and therapy, the Conductor. The Conductor works with the help of assistants and employs the technique of 'rhythmic intention'. Rhythmic intention is based on the proposition that behaviour can be regulated or controlled through verbalisation of the activity. Thus, client and Conductor verbalise the movement being undertaken and rhythmically count as it is undertaken. During the exercise of a movement in this way, Peto emphasised that the client should not be touched. The function of working in groups is to enhance motivation through both competition and mutual support.

Though Cotton and Parnwell (1968) claim impressive results with a group of athetoid children in a modified version of the Peto method, research with a group of children who were profoundly retarded and multiply impaired leads to a less optimistic conclusion with respect to this population. Cottam, McCartney and Cullen (1985) studied ten such children of 4 years of age and over, splitting them into two groups of five, only one group receiving conductive education. Teaching based on this method was carried out for 22 months for 25 minutes per day around the activities of eating and drinking. No significant improvement relative to the control group (who received conventional behavioural programmes) was noted in any of the areas of sitting balance, attentional control, object permanence, co-operation with an adult, receptive language, vocal and motor imitation, symbolic play, self-help skills and independence. It should be noted that teachers employing the techniques did, however, themselves consider that improvement had taken place.

Failure of conductive education with this group may reflect the fact that the technique was not implemented with the intensity advocated by Peto and his followers. On the other hand, a relatively high level of functioning is assumed by the requirement of rhythmic intention that behaviour can be regulated by language. Indeed, with respect to both conductive education and co-active therapy, limitations may be placed on the effectiveness of the approaches by the important part played by verbal comprehension.

Sensorimotor Patterning. Intensity of treatment is also an element in the application of sensorimotor patterning that has become known as the 'Doman-Delacato Technique' to which we have drawn attention in Chapter 2. Doman and Delacato's work had been developed for a quarter of a century in the Institutes for the Achievement of Human Potential (IAHP) in Philadelphia. A significant breakaway group established the American Academy for Human Development (AAHD), employing procedures from other therapies in addition to the methods evolved by Doman and Delacato. In the UK, related organisations linked in different degrees to IAHP have been established.

The theoretical basis for this approach has been summarised by LeWinn, Doman, Delacato, Spitz and Thomas (1966):

> The process of learning is dependent upon the complexity of development and organization of the central nervous system. The development of the central nervous system depends upon its opportunities to take in and react to the stimuli offered by its environment. Variations in environmental stimulation result in variations in the ability to learn. Sensory deprivation and, therefore, lack of expressive opportunity for reinforcement can be the result of environmental variations. However, sensory deprivation and lack of expressive opportunity for reinforcement can also result from trauma to the central nervous system. Because of such trauma the central nervous system may be unable to react either at a receptive or an expressive level. (p. 53)

The damaged brain will not learn with normal environmental input and requires increased stimulation in frequency, intensity and duration. Conventional approaches to the effects of brain damage, it is claimed, emphasise systems, not therapy that will directly affect the pathological condition of the brain. In terms of symptoms, brain damage will affect the chronological age at which functioning is achieved in the six areas defined as central in the approach, walking, talking, writing, reading, understanding speech and stereognosis (all assessable using the Doman-Delacato Developmental profile). The achievement of such functions is considered significant because it reflects the *Neurological Age* of the child which in turn reflects the degree of neurological organisation and hence the functional capacity of the brain.

This theoretical position leads to the argument that treatment of brain damage should be just that, not symptomatic treatment of the consequences of the pathology. Five treatment principles are then derived:

(i)   Procedures which supply basic discrete bits of information to the brain for storage: this intervention is entirely sensory in nature and involves stimulation of all modalities — auditory, visual, tactile, taste, smell, etc.

(ii)   Procedures which programme the brain itself. Here the patterning techniques associated with the Doman-Delacato method are employed. The intention is that sensory input is given in the form of motor patterns that eventually will be the basis for voluntary movement. The sequence is critical following what is regarded as a biologically determined order. It begins with child lying prone and movements of head and trunk; in the same position, homolateral movement patterns are carried out, i.e. the arm and leg on the side the child is facing are flexed and on the other side are extended; contralateral patterning follows with the arm on the face side flexed and the leg extended, arm and leg in opposite flexion-extension on the other side of the body; reciprocal crawling on hands and knees follows after which walking is patterned. Patterning procedures for hand movements are also undertaken.

(iii) Techniques are employed to induce actual movements in relation to specific stimuli.

(iv)   Acquired patterns of movement are encouraged as voluntary activities.

(v)   Attempts to improve the physiological environment are carried out, notably increasing the blood flow to the head through inhalation of CO_2.

Proponents of this approach have presented their own evidence for the effectiveness of their techniques with a wide range of pathologies. Independent evaluation is limited, however, though Newman, Roos, McCann, Menolascino and Heal (1974) present positive evidence with young people who were severely to moderately retarded with respect to improvement in visual perception, mobility and language. This study was undertaken on the breakaway AAHD programme and we are not aware of comparable evaluations of the IAHP programme in relation to individuals who are profoundly retarded and multiply impaired.

Neurodevelopment Treatment with Reflex Inhibition and Facilitation: The Bobath Method. Of the 'named' approaches we have reviewed so far, the approach of K. and B. Bobath is most specifically directed to physical impairment in general and cerebral palsy in particular. Bobath (1966) describes the theoretical basis for the therapy advocated. He indicates that motor development is characterised by two sets of processes which are closely interwoven: (i) development of normal postural reflex mechanisms that are associated with normal postural tone, maintenance of position and performance of normal movements; and (ii) inhibition of some neonatal responses, e.g. primary standing and walking.

> This process, sometimes referred to as 'breaking up' of the early total responses, makes possible re-synthesis of parts of the total patterns in many and varied ways, and, in association with the development of as normal postural reflex mechanism ... allows for the performance of selective movements such as walking and especially for the perfection of manipulative skills. (p. 1)

In cerebral palsy the lesion interferes with this orderly development leading to: (i) inadequate postural reflex mechanisms; and (ii) unduly long prolongation of primitive patterns. Abnormal postures and movements will result and will be incompatible with normal motor behaviour. *Primitive* motor behaviour refers to persistence of normal full-term babies' patterns of movement and posture and 'abnormal' refers to patterns of movement and posture not seen at any time in babies' post-natal life.

Treatment is based on the answer to three questions: What makes the client assume an abnormal posture? Which are the recurring patterns of muscle function in posture and movement that make selective movements impossible? Which basic automatic movements are missing? (Bobath 1955 p. 151).

> The treatment is based on the idea that the teaching of normal movements and the correction of postures is impossible as long as the muscle tone in abnormal and released tonic reflexes are present. Before the patient can be expected to have normal coordination in voluntary movements and skills, we have to help him to inhibit his abnormal posture and movement reactions, and we have to develop such automatic movements as righting reflexes and equilibrium reactions. (p. 51)

Abnormal postural reflex activity is inhibited through a special technique of manipulation, i.e. reflex-inhibiting postures. Automatic movements such as righting reflexes are facilitated. Spontaneous movements are induced by moving clients into position. Bobath argues that normal automatic movements are under control in an adequate reflex inhibiting posture.

Bobath (1967) has emphasised the importance of early intervention, i.e. before 9 months of age, in order to capitalise on the plasticity of the infant brain and encourage sensorimotor learning and prevent compounding of mental handicap. In addition, abnormal postural patterns are usually weaker in the infant and are therefore more modifiable. At this stage, too, contractures and deformities can be avoided and more rapid results achieved.

The clear theoretical statement underlying the Bobath's approach and its grounding in neurophysiology should not blind us to the fact that the aim of their treatment is quite explicitly to permit ultimately the development of skilled movement for everyday life and self-help activities (Bobath 1963).

The Eclectic Viewpoint. The reader will now have some idea of the basis for the more prominent 'named' approaches in this area. While he or she will on occasions encounter proponents of these positions, it is more likely that the physiotherapist with whom he or she collaborates will have taken something from each approach, and indeed others we have not dealt with here. Such selection is referred to by Levitt (1982) as the 'Eclectic viewpoint in therapy', and it is the position she herself adopts, arguing that there is much common ground between the theories and even common practice where theory differs. While acknowledging that there are differences in method and rationale, central to all approaches is a concern with:

(i)   Postural Mechanisms: These include: (a) The antigravity mechanisms such as the 'supporting reaction' in infants. (b) Postural fixation of parts of the body, i.e. stability. (c) Counterpoising mechanisms-adjustments while maintaining posture, balance during motion; (d) Righting or rising reaction, assumption of posture when, for example, standing or sitting. (e) Tilt reaction — self righting. (f) Reaction to falling or saving from fall-protective extension of limbs. Levitt indicates that these postural reactions are stimulated or trained in all systems of therapy, though with different reactions emphasised in different systems.

(ii)   Voluntary Motion: Involves many different synergies and is dependent upon postural mechanisms to provide a base from which to move. Underlying voluntary motion are a variety of other perceptual and cognitive processes.

(iii)   Perceptual-motor Functioning: Linking of sensations and sensory discrimination are central to the activites of physio, speech and occupational therapy. From this common ground Levitt argues for treatment principles based on a synthesis of the various therapy systems. The general principles that inform this system are team work, early treatment, repetition of a motor activity (by session and on day-long basis), sensory motor experience for and motivation of the client.

Specific principles relate to:

(i)   Developmental Training: It is insufficient to advocate 'normal motor developmental sequences'. Decisions have to be taken on what the units of the total motor function are that need to be trained and different positions vary on this. Levitt argues that, nevertheless, all levels of analysis are relevant from work on gross patterns, e.g. sensorimotor patterning, through to work on individual muscles and their tone. Strict sequencing of objectives is only relevant within a specific target, e.g. independent head control, not between different 'milestone' objectives. Where necessary, sequences should be modified to suit the individual client. The developmental view adopted by Levitt is that several motor functions evolve in parallel, e.g. mechanisms relevant to walking are developed along with those leading to independent sitting. She 'uses parallel developmental sequences with selected motor activities which are fundamental postural reactions' (p. 40). In her practical chapters she selects ideas from various approaches to train motor activities in developmental sequences.

(ii)   Treatment of Abnormal Tone: Levitt points out that it is not spasticity in itself that prevents the development of voluntary movement; postural control is more important and is independent of spasticity. Where spasticity is relevant to function is when it contributes to abnormal posture or deformities which present a mechanical block to function. Hypotonicity is apparently not associated with strength of voluntary movements but with postural reactions. Where tone is fluctuating the relation to postural control is not clear, but training seems to decrease disrupting effects of spasm and sometimes degree of involuntary motion.

(iii)   Training of Movement Patterns: It is *generally* advisable to 'stimulate movements initially through synkinetic movements, then modify these primitive combinations of movements into more controlled and advanced patterns and finally into selective or isolated movements' (Levitt 1982 p. 44).

(iv)   Use of Afferent Stimuli: Afferent input by the therapist through touch, pressure, resisted motion, joint compression, input of visual and auditory stimuli gives the child the experience of movement that cannot be attained voluntarily. This can be taken over consciously, but muscle actions, movements synergies and postures become unconscious and involuntary after they have been achieved. At the appropriate level of language comprehension, language input can also be employed as advocated by Peto, though we have already noted above the limitations of such an approach where profound retardation is present.

(v)   Passive or Active Motion: Levitt makes the important point that: 'Passive 'patterning' of children or a 'full range of passive motion' cannot contribute much, if anything, to training motion. They can only keep the joints mobile, and help to prevent deformity' (p. 46). Active or active resisted motion provides better proprioceptive information than passive movement alone.

(vi)   Facilitation: Abnormal and normal 'overflow' can be facilitated by the therapist. 'Any patterns facilitated in one part of the body should be accompanied by careful observation of the whole child and not only of the part being activated. Normal or abnormal 'overflow' of motor activity should be observed when using techniques in one part of the body to facilitate activity in other parts of the body' (Levitt 1982 p. 47).

(vii)   Prevention of Deformity: This can be caused by a variety of factors, Hare (1975) lists unequal pull of spastic muscles, persistence of tonic neck reflexes, inappropriate, prolonged posture and support. An inability to move underlies all these causes. Common deformities include subluxation of the hips, scoliosis with distortion of the rib cage, contratures of flexors of neck, elbow, hip, knee and Achilles' tendon. Positioning of the client throughout the day and use of appropriate prosthetics are critical activities for all caregivers of people who are profoundly retarded and immobile as a result of physical impairment. A detailed account of approaches to positioning to avoid deformities is given by Levitt (1982 Chapter 8).

Levitt (1982) also draws attention to the special needs of the visually impaired child (see also for a general account of the physiotherapists input to the visually impaired child Sykanda and Levitt 1982). She notes that lack of a visual frame of reference leads to poor posture and hypotonia. Special training is required using auditory, tactile, proprioceptive and vestibular stimuli. The importance of developing hand function is also described. Suggestions for the development of hand function in blind cerebral palsied children are often based on a general account of hand function development (pp. 172–93). Levitt's discussion draws attention to the important point that individuals who are profoundly retarded and have a visual, but not specific motor, impairment, nevertheless require attention with respect to motor function.

In addition to the gross motor functioning outlined above, direct attention to hand function in people who are profoundly retarded and physically and/or visually impaired, will be central to intervention. Levitt points out that hand function must be considered in relation to motor control of the shoulder girdle, arms and hands, as well as visual, perceptual, perceptual-motor and cognitive development. Postural fixation of the shoulder girdle helps reach, reach and grasp and co-ordinated manipulation. Head, trunk and pelvic postural fixation and counterpoising in sitting and standing permit hand use in other than lying. Abnormal functioning of the upper limbs is also a target of remediation in its own right. Both Holle (1976) and Levitt (1982) offer a wealth of practical information on the development of hand function.

Two further issues require comment with respect to teachers and other caregivers providing an appropriate 'motor environment' for profoundly retarded physically impaired individuals. These are handling and the use of aids.

With respect to handling, several excellent and well-illustrated manuals are available. Finnie (1974) describes (Chapter 4) how control of abnormal patterns in individuals with cerebral palsy can be effected by giving support at *key points*. These are the head, neck, spine, shoulder, shoulder girdle, hips and pelvis. She presents 15 pages (pp. 53–67) of detailed figures that are essential study for teachers and other caregivers and will assist in interpreting the advice and demonstrations of physiotherapists. The approach to handling begins with the initial contact with child. Sensitivity in making this initial contact is emphasised by

McInnes and Treffry (1982) and is clearly of special importance where
the person is visually impaired and whose first knowledge that he or
she is about to be moved may be tactile. Sensitivity during holding is
also urged by Finnie:

> To do this successfully you will need to learn, with the help of your
> therapist, to observe and to understand the reasons for your child's
> difficulties in moving and how these vary, to be aware how his
> abnormal patterns of posture and movement affect the whole body,
> and how by handling at 'key-points' you can influence or change these
> reactions. During treatment sessions your therapist will demonstrate
> and teach you the techniques that can be used to inhibit or increase
> muscle tone in appropriate cases, and how to combine special techni-
> ques of inhibition with facilitation. (p. 52)

Law and Suckling (1983) also provide a well-illustrated guide to
handling which deals among other topics with respiration (including
postural drainage, sucking, swallowing, coughing and air swallowing)
and sleeping.

A range of appliances and aids are available for, and essential to,
individuals who are profoundly retarded and multiply impaired. They
range from basic seating and gross support systems, to prosthetics for
specific limbs, through to microelectronic devices that give feedback of
motor function. Decisions on the use of such aids will rest partly with
the caregiver and will usually require consultation with the
physiotherapist. A detailed listing of relevant material is beyond the scope
of this book, but the reader is referred to Barton, Holloborn and Woods
(1980) to an evaluation of aids and appliances for children with handicaps
which is accompanied by a useful list of catalogues and suppliers. Levitt
(1982) concludes her own book with a detailed appendix on equipment
and a list of addresses of organisations with whom consultation can be
undertaken. Finnie (1974) presents a chapter on prams, pushchairs and
chairs (Chapter 12) from which we will limit ourselves to a quotation
on bean bags:

> *Please note* that we *do not recommend* the use of this chair for the
> very inactive, floppy or flexed child. We repeat *only* use this chair
> for the severely extended handicapped child who is unable to learn
> any form of postural control and then *only* for short periods. (p. 159).

Other chapters in this book deal with hammocks, wedges and prone boards (Chapter 13) and aids to mobility (Chapter 14).

The synthesis of the specific physiotherapeutic procedures, including handling techniques and use of aids, will result in a comprehensive programme for an individual person. This will be integrated with a variety of other curricular and day to day activities and indeed will be pointed ultimately to providing a basis for successful adaptive behaviour. Levitt (1982) notes how such a programme leads into improved motor function in feeding, dressing, toileting, washing, bathing, play and communication.

The activities of physiotherapists and their colleagues are undertaken daily in a variety of facilities but are rarely reported in a book or article form as comprehensive programmes. Several examples of such programmes do exist, however, some aimed at improving motor dysfunction, some at enhancing development in its own right, and others concerned with both. Of those dealing explicity with people with profound retardation we will describe the following two programmes, the first concerned with development, the second with dysfunction.

The Gross Motor Programme of Alter, Goldstein and Molnar (1983). Alter *et al.*'s programme is directed to individuals who are severely and profoundly retarded but without obvious neurological damage. It is of interest because it is conceived as part of a total *Social Learning Curriculum*. Within this wider curriculum the Gross Motor Programme is viewed as establishing functional strategies to mediate environmental interactions. Movement will permit the student to acquire new information and to enhance responsiveness to other people. Theoretically the programme is rooted in neurophysiological studies and emphasises the importance of postural control in the development of motor behaviour (see Molnar 1978, discussed in Volume 1, Chapter 3, p. 82). It focuses on the acquisition of motor skills across the whole spectrum on the basis of the body positions of lying, sitting and moving about. Instructional strategies are laid down with step-by-step information on how the intervention should be conducted.

Auxter's Gross Motor Development Programme (Auxter 1971). In contrast, Auxter's programme is directed to people who are profoundly retarded and have clear impairment to movement (in his own work of Chronological Age (CA) 12 to 30 years and Mental Age (MA) 6 to 18 months). It focuses on four key areas, increasing range of motion, development of extensor strength, proprioceptive stimulation and development of integrative function of the joints.

Developing Specific Motor Programmes. Both Alter *et al.* and Auxter's programmes directly invoke the principles of applied behaviour analysis or behaviour modification in implementing them. Levitt (1982), too, argues that such implementation by a physiotherapist should be informed by a knowledge of learning principles (pp. 20–3). One implication of this view is that specific motor targets within the wider programme may be dealt with as behavioural programmes in their own right, particularly when they constitute areas of particular concern. Below we list and offer brief summaries of some published studies as models for the development of such intervention, concentrating on head control, sitting and mobility, and the use of hands and arms.

Some Specific Studies

We have discussed in Chapter 2 (p. 49ff.) the development of behavioural teaching techniques and programmes and such procedures in the area of motor development and competence are highly applicable. Motor behaviours are generally readily observable and amenable to physical shaping. In our own experience, however, it is neither economical nor productive to attempt to teach all motor skills in a formal trial-by-trial fashion. Walking on a bar to improve balance can be fun for a limited period of time as a game, but becomes boring and ineffective if repeated ten or twenty times towards some preset criterion. Judgement needs to be exercised, therefore, as to when it is useful and productive to set out a formal behavioural programme and implement it as a priority. In other instances objectives can be incorporated into wider activities which encourage motor development.

In order to illustrate some of the features of specific programmes we describe briefly some that have been employed with people who are profoundly retarded, usually individuals with additional impairments. We cover head control, aspects of sitting and ambulation, including the goal directed use of ambulation to get from one place to another. Aspects of arm and hand function ranging from reaching to grasp are then considered.

Head Control. Sebba (1978), working with a group of preschool children who are profoundly retarded and have additional impairments, describes several programmes dealing with aspects of head control. For child ZP, for example, an objective of head raising in prone was set. No prompting was employed and reinforcement was auditory, a rattle waved in front of the child who was visually impaired. Employing short sessions of five trials, a criterion of four successive days on which ZP held her head up for 20 seconds or more was achieved in 49 sessions. Head raising in prone was also undertaken with child MM who was physically impaired but sighted. Here, following the instruction: 'Head up, M!', music and 'Good boy!', were employed as reinforcers. A more stringent objective of 60 seconds or more for five sessions was set and achieved after 69, three-minute sessions. A programme of head raising in supine was also initiated with this child but abandoned in favour of head control during a pull-to-sit programme which we describe below.

With the children in Sebba's programme, head control in lying position was taught. Such techniques can readily be extended to children who are sitting but have poor head control. Approaches to establishing head control in children who are physically and mentally handicapped are described by Grove, Dalke, Fredericks and Crowley (1975). The possibility of utilising electronics or microelectronics to provide feedback or reinforcement has increasingly become an option. Ball, McCrady and Hart (1975) describe how a transistor radio was activated by a mercury switch to reinforce head posture in two children who were retarded and had cerebral palsy. Under the contigent music condition, dropping the head forward automatically terminated the broadcast music, leading to marked improvements in head posture.

Sitting. While the possibility of appropriate positioning of an individual in a sitting posture must be considered, programmed movement towards independent maintenance of sitting posture is a central curricular aim. Sebba (1978) describes several programmes related to different aspects of sitting. ZP was taught to improve her pull-to-sit behaviour though some prompting remained necessary and the objective of five unprompted responses on each of five days was not achieved. MM also was placed on a programme of pull to sit with the aim of encouraging head control as he was raised, i.e. that during the lift his head should not lag behind. HJ was taught to get into a sitting posture from supine with beads being employed as both prompt and reinforcement. Thirty-eight half-hour sessions were required for the criterion of ten unprompted responses to be achieved successfully on each of five days. Though ZP failed to pull to sit during the course of the programme, she did attain independent sitting in a programme in which whistles and horns were employed as reinforcers. The criterion of independent sitting for more than 40 seconds on each of five consecutive days was achieved in 48 sessions of 10 trials each.

Ambulation. A variety of successful programmes teaching walking to children and adults who are profoundly retarded have been reported. This activity is clearly central to all therapy-based accounts cited above and general statements on what has to be taken into account in developing such programmes for individuals who are retarded are available (e.g. Wilson and Parks 1970). Loynd and Barclay (1970) taught walking to an 8 year old child who was microcephalic and profoundly retarded. This child could stand and take a few steps while grasping tables. Independent movement was taught by reinforcing the child for moving between two tables using a broom handle resting between them and for walking towards the therapist. With progress in this direction, a dowel was used, held by therapist and child, for holding as the child walked. This was faded to a short stick, to a piece of tape, to a piece of string. Finally independent walking with minimal support from the string was achieved. In addition to independent mobility the authors of this article note improvements in both social and communicative behaviour.

Feldstein and Girouard (1983) report what they claim is the first published study on walking with an adult who was profoundly retarded. She was 27 years of age with no language and required assistance in all self-help skills. She had poor vision, some hearing loss and abnormalities of both knees. She moved by bottom-scooting but would walk if her hand was held. The procedure employed involved response priming, prevention of inappropriate responding, fading of support and reinforcement for walking. Backward chaining was employed with the client one step from a table on which a fruit drink stood. Forward movement was prevented if the client dropped and tried to scoot forward. The distance from the table was progressively lengthened to over 4 metres. In the second phase, self-initiated walking in several regularly encountered settings was taught and progress to independent walking without scooting was achieved with support from other staff. Some prompting was, however, required and reversions to scooting did occur. The extension to the more complex ambulation skill of stair climbing has also been reported Cipani (1982).

The move into familiar settings in Feldstein and Girouard's study emphasises the fact that walking is not an end in itself but a means to enable the client to move freely in his or her environment. What has been referred to as 'route travel' has been taught in a limited number of studies. Sebba (1978 p. 204) notes a programme for a child who could crawl but bumped into objects. Here the route to be traversed was simply to crawl beneath a table leaf without coming into contact with any part of the table. At the other extreme Gruber, Reeser and Reid (1979) set out to teach the use of walking skills to adults who were profoundly retarded (IQs 8, 9, 11 and 14). They were able to respond to simple commands and were ambulant. A complex training programme was initiated which resulted in all four clients learning to walk from their ward to the residential school on request and independently.

Where visual impairment exists, then some form of tactile or auditory cueing will be necessary for such independent mobility to be achieved. Uslan, Malone and De L'Aune (1983) developed a novel approach to this problem with a group of adult clients that included individuals who were profoundly retarded and blind. Each specific location in their residence was associated with a particular piece of music, e.g. the women's toilet with 'I am a Woman' and the counselling room with 'Amazing Grace'. Routes to each room had speakers that came on successively playing the relevant piece of music. These were switched on by under floor contacts as the resident walked along the route. Successful following of the music to the target room was achieved by all clients, though it does appear that when the music was faded out it may not have been possible for individuals with profound retardation to continue this success, perhaps because of a failure to develop a spatial map associated with their own bodily movement.

Feldstein and Girouard's study also draws attention to the occasional need to eliminate inappropriate ways of moving round in order to ensure ambulation. O'Brien, Azrin and Bugle (1972) report a similar study with four children with profound retardation who crawled in preference to walking. A restraint procedure was used in which the child was held for five seconds if he or she attempted to crawl. Walking was primed by lifting the children onto their feet. All four children shifted to walking as the preferred mobility strategy and the programme was implemented by nursery staff and required no special apparatus.

In addition to the development of route travel as an ultimate end of teaching ambulation, consideration must also be given to wider aspects of mobility related to leisure. Participation in sport and dance are both suitable long-term goals for many individuals who are profoundly retarded. Specific programmes are now being evolved and Lagomarcino, Reid, Ivancic and Faw (1984) report one such study in which leisure-dance activities were taught and employed acceptably in a community setting with some support from their caregivers.

Upper Limb Functions. The importance of reach and grasp activities in development has already been made clear in earlier discussions of sensorimotor activities. For that reason, much of this topic has been dealt with in Chapter 3. Correa, Poulson and Salzberg (1984) report on teaching reach and grasp to children who were blind and retarded. Similarly, much of what was written about 'simple' operant conditioning involved upper limb activities as in the case of Fuller's (1949) study. Certainly any effective programme directed at upper limb activity will result in sensorimotor gains as they increase the range of schemes and their co-ordination.

Reach and grasp behaviours can in some instances be considered separately for programming purposes. Thus Sebba (1978) describes two programmes for child SA, one concerned with grasp and the other with reaching. The former required SA to grasp her father's finger for a count of 20 with social and edible reinforcement and the use of physical prompting. This was achieved in 69 sessions, the behaviour generalising to a held peg. Arm raising to a rod 15 inches above the floor was also taught in the same way, criterion being achieved in 15 sessions.

Continued grasping was taught by Jones (1980) to a 13 year old girl who was cortically blind and had spasticity of both legs. Objects were placed in her hands and contingent vibratory reinforcement employed. She progressed not only to holding objects but searching for, shaking, lifting and exploring them — particularly music-producing toys. She went on to hold and use a spoon during mealtimes. Clearly, once grasping of objects had been achieved, the way was opened to her to exercise a variety of sensorimotor schemes related to objects.

Arm movement was central to both the Sebba programme noted above and to other programmes developed in the light of Fuller's (1949) study. Murphy and Doughty (1977), working with seven children who were profoundly retarded and cerebral palsied, taught a behaviour requiring pulling a weighted cord, either up or down, vibration again being the contingency. Demands were increased with respect to both the actual weight pulled and the extent to which the cord has to be grasped rather than looped round the wrist. Success was achieved in this programme and the authors note its relevance to physical therapy and education.

Motor Competence

Many of the programmes described lead to the convergence of motor and cognitive behaviour, and throughout have been concerned to emphasise motor development and the overcoming of dysfunction as means to adaptive behaviour in real-life settings. Adaptive behaviour is the outcome of the successful execution of goals set by or for an individual. Motor competence refers to the capacity to realise such goals through motor activity appropriate to the particular end in view. Such competence, of course, is not dependent upon motor function alone, but rests too on cognitive development that permits goal planning.

Elsewhere we have discussed in detail the implication of this view of motor competence for the curriculum for individuals who are retarded (Hogg 1986). This position is equally applicable to individuals with profound retardation and multiple impairment. Where prerequisite motor and cognitive behaviours have been established, or where motor dysfunction can be circumvented by suitable prosthetics, such individuals can move into programmes that enhance adaptive behaviour in both self-help and leisure activities. The overall framework for implementing such programmes will remain the same as that described in Hogg (1986). Objectives will be defined with respect to the activity itself and the situations to which it must generalise. Detailed tasks analysis will specify not only the training steps involved but also the co-ordination of teaching methods within the overall programme. While the special needs of people with profound retardation and multiple impairments will always require careful consideration of techniques specific to their needs, with the move into considering motor competence as a curricular area we find that the strategies applicable to more able people with retardation become increasingly relevant.

References

Almond, S. (1982) 'The Role of the Physiotherapist' in C. Gunstone, J. Hogg, J. Sebba, J. Warner and S. Almond (eds.), *Classroom Provision and Organisation for Integrated Preschool Children*, Barnardos Publications Ltd, Barkingside

Alter, M., Goldstein, H. and Molnar, G.E. (1983) 'Development of a Gross Motor Programme in Educational Curriculum for Severely Retarded Students: A Transdisciplinary Approach' in J. Hogg and P. Mittler (eds.), *Advances in Mental Handicap Research: Vol. 2, Aspects of Competence in Mentally Handicapped People*, Wiley, Chichester

Auxter, D. (1971) 'Motor Skill Development in the Profoundly Retarded', *Training School Bulletin, 68*, 5–9

Ball, T.S., McCrady, R.E. and Hart, A.D. (1975) 'Automated Reinforcement of Head Posture in Two Cerebral Palsied Retarded Children', *Perceptual and Motor Skills, 40*, 619–22

Barton, E.M., Holloborn, B. and Woods, G.E. (1980) 'Appliances Used to Help the Handicapped Under Threes to Follow the Normal Developmental Sequence', *Child: Care, Health and Development, 6,* 209–32

Bayley, N. (1969) *Scales of Infant Development,* Psychological Corporation, New York

Bobath, B. (1955) 'The Treatment of Motor Disorders of Pyramidal and Extra-pyramidal Origin by Reflex Inhibition and by Facilitation of Movement', *Physiotherapy, 41,* 146–53

Bobath, B. (1963) 'Treatment Principles and Planning in Cerebral Palsy', *Physiotherapy, 49,* 122–4

Bobath, B. (1967) 'The Very Early Treatment of Cerebral Palsy', *Developmental Medicine and Child Neurology, 9,* 373–90

Bobath, K. (1966) 'The Motor Deficit in Patients with Cerebral Palsy', *Clinics in Developmental Medicine, 23,* Heinemann, London

Cipani, E. (1982) 'Teaching Profoundly Retarded Adults to Ascend Stairs Safely', *Education and Training of the Mentally Retarded, 17,* 51–4

Correa, V.I., Poulson, C.L. and Salzberg, C.L. (1984) 'Training and Generalization of Reach-Grasp Behavior in Blind, Retarded Young Children', *Journal of Applied Behavior Analysis, 17,* 57–69

Cottam, P., McCartney, E. and Cullen, C. (1985) 'The Effectiveness of Conductive Education Principles with Profoundly Retarded Multiply Handicapped Children', *British Journal of Disorders of Communication, 20,* 45–60

Cottam, P. and Sutton, A. (eds.) (1985) *Conductive Education: A System for Overcoming Motor Disorder,* Croom Helm, London, Sydney and Dover, N.H.

Cotton, E. (1965) 'The Institute of Movement Therapy and School for Conductors: A Report of a Study Visit', *Developmental Medicine and Child Neurology, 7,* 437–46

Cotton, E. and Parnwell, M. (1968) 'Conductive Education with Special Reference to Severe Athetoids in a Non-residential Centre', *Journal of Mental Subnormality, 14,* 50–6

Feldstein, J.H. and Girouard, M. (1983) 'Development of Independent Walking in a Profoundly Retarded Woman', *Psychological Reports, 52,* 563–8

Finnie, N. (1974) *Handling the Young Cerebral Palsied Child at Home,* Heinemann, London

Fuller, P.R. (1949) 'Operant Conditioning of a Vegetative Human Organism', *American Journal of Psychology, 62,* 587–90

Griffiths, R. (1970) *Griffiths Mental Development Scales,* Child Development Research Centre, Taunton

Grove, N.D., Dalke, B.A., Fredericks, H.D. and Crowley, R.F. (1975) 'Establishing Appropriate Head Positioning with Mentally and Physically Handicapped Children', *Behavioral Engineering, 3,* 53–9

Gruber, B., Reeser, R. and Reid, D.H. (1979) 'Providing a Less Restrictive Environment for Profoundly Retarded Persons by Teaching Independent Skills', *Journal of Applied Behavior Analysis, 12,* 285–97

Guess, D., Rues, J., Warren, S., Lyon, S., Mulligan, M., Lehr, D., Janssen, C., Murphy, N., Fosage, K. and Barnes, K. (1979) 'Assessment of Motor and Sensory/Motor Acquisition in Handicapped and Nonhandicapped Infants and Young Children [ECI Document Number 126]', University of Kansas

Gunstone, C. (1979, revised 1985) *Checklists used at Anson House Preschool Project* Dr Barnardo's Publications, Barkingside

Hare, N. (1975) 'Physiotherapy' in Kirman, B. and Bicknell, J. (eds.), *Mental Handicap,* Churchill Livingstone, London

Hogg, J. (1986) 'Motor Competence in Children with Mental Handicap' J. Coupe and J. Porter (eds.), *The Education of Children with Severe Learning Difficulties: Bridging the Gap Between Theory and Practice,* Croom Helm, London

Holle, B. (1976) *Motor Development in Children: Normal and Retarded,* Blackwell, London

Hollis, K. (1977a) *Progress to Movement: For Mentally Handicapped Children and Adults with Additional Physical Handicap,* Institute of Mental Subnormality, Kidderminster

Hollis, K. (1977b) *Progress to Standing: For Children with Severe Physical and Mental Handicap,* Institute of Mental Subnormality, Kidderminster

Jones, C. (1980) 'The Uses of Mechanical Vibration with the Severely Mentally Handicapped. Part II: Behavioural Effects', *Apex, 7,* 112–14

Lagomarcino, A., Reid, D.H., Ivancic, M.T. and Faw, G.D. (1984) 'Leisure-dance Instruction for Severely and Profoundly Retarded Persons: Teaching an Intermediate Community Living Skill', *Journal of Applied Behavior Analysis, 17,* 71–84

Law, I.H. and Suckling, M.H. (1983) *Handling when Children are Profoundly Handicapped,* Jordanhill College of Education, Glasgow

Levitt, S. (1982) *Treatment of Cerebral Palsy and Motor Delay,* 2nd edn, Blackwell Scientific Publishers, Oxford

LeWinn, E.B., Doman, G., Delacato, C.H., Spitz, E.B. and Thomas, E.W. (1966) 'Neurological Organization: The Basis for Learning' in J. Hellmuth (ed.), *Learning Disorders: Vol. 2,* Special Child Publications, Seattle

Loynd, J. and Barclay, A. (1970) 'A Case Study in Developing Ambulation in a Profoundly Retarded Child', *Behaviour Research and Therapy, 8,* 207

McInnes, J.M. and Treffry, J.A. (1982) *Deaf-Blind Infants and Children: A Developmental Guide,* University of Toronto Press, Toronto/Open University Press, Milton Keynes

Mira, M. (1977) 'Tracking the Motor Behavior Development of Multihandicapped Infants', *Mental Retardation, 15,* 32–7

Murphy, R.J. and Doughty, N.R. (1977) 'Establishment of Controlled Arm Movement in Profoundly Retarded Students Using Response Contingent Vibratory Stimulation', *American Journal of Mental Deficiency, 82,* 212–16

Newman, R., Roos, P., McCann, B.M., Menolascino, F.J. and Heal, L.W. (1974) 'Experimental Evaluation of Sensorimotor Patterning Used with Mentally Retarded Children', *American Journal of Mental Deficiency, 79,* 372–84

O'Brien, F., Azrin, N.H. and Bugle, C. (1972) 'Training Profoundly Retarded Children to Stop Crawling', *Journal of Applied Behavior Analysis, 5,* 131–7

Sebba, J. (1978) 'A System for Assessment and Intervention for Preschool Profoundly Retarded Multiply Handicapped Children', unpublished M.Ed. thesis, University of Manchester, Manchester

Shearer, M.S. and Shearer, D. (1972) 'The Portage Project: A Model for Early Childhood Education', *Exceptional Children, 39,* 210–17

Sykanda, A.M. and Levitt, S. (1982) 'The Physiotherapist in the Developmental

Management of the Visually Impaired Child', *Child Care, Health and Development, 8,* 261–70

Tomporowski, P.D. and Ellis, N.R. (1984) 'Preparing Severely and Profoundly Mentally Retarded Adults for Tests of Motor Fitness', *Adapted Physical Activity Quarterly, 1,* 158–63

Uslan, M., Malone, S., and De l'Aune, W. (1983) 'Teaching Route Travel to Multiply Handicapped Blind Adults: An Auditory Approach', *Journal of Visual Impairment and Blindness,* January, 18–20

Van Dijk, J. (1977) 'What We Have Learned in Twelve and a Half Years: Principles of Deaf-blind Education' in M.R. Jurgens (ed.), *Confrontation between the Young Deaf-Blind Child and the Outer World,* Swets and Zeitlinger, Lisse

Wilson, V. and Parks, R. (1970) 'Promoting Ambulation in the Severely Retarded Child', *Mental Retardation, 8,* 17–19

6 SELF-HELP SKILLS

Introduction

Self-help skills along with cognitive skills, communication and motor skills, are considered priority areas for people with profound retardation and multiple impairments by parents and professionals alike. Hence, this provides the focus for the final chapter on the specific curricular areas covered in this book. The reader will recall that in Volume 1, Chapter 1 we noted the low level of self-help skills associated with profound retardation and multiple impairment. This population was characterised in our functional definitions as often doubly incontinent and unable to feed or dress themselves.

It is clear that the recent trend towards deinstitutionalisation makes it all the more essential for people to have these basic everyday skills, without which they are likely to be the last to leave or only people remaining, within the institutions. It is probable that their lack of adequate feeding and toileting skills combined with their frequency of behaviour problems, discussed in the next chapter, makes this the population least likely to attract staff. Moreover, the very high proportion of time spent by staff and clients conducting these basic daily essentials leaves little time for the other varied activities which, we hope we have clearly stated earlier in this book, can be beneficial to this population. Balthazar, Naor and Sindberg (1973) have shown that in the absence of training programmes people with profound impairments show no spontaneous improvement in self-help skills. Studies over the last 20 years (e.g. Bensberg, Colwell and Cassell 1965) have demonstrated that these skills can improve when intervention does take place. Most importantly, the self-dignity and control over their own environment which people can experience when they are no longer dependent on others for every basic need, is perhaps the fundamental reason for giving high priority to the teaching of self-help skills.

The definition of what to include within the area of self-help skills is somewhat arbitrary, as was noted in Chapter 2 of this volume in relation to every area of the curriculum. All curricular materials reviewed in Chapter 2 included self-help skills in some form although under a variety of names such as daily living skills, independence skills, etc. Most of these covered at least toilet training, feeding and dressing. Many cover, in addition, more advanced skills such as grooming (hairdressing, shaving), cooking, shopping and sewing. For the population we have defined as having profound retardation and multiple impairments, the skills involved in using the toilet, dressing and eating probably provide sufficient scope for teaching programmes. However, as McInnes and Treffry (1982) point out the person who has multiple impairments but not profound retardation should not be limited to these skills. They suggest that the child with hearing and visual impairments must also be taught to shop, purchase and care for clothes, use public transport, etc. These authors provide clear and useful suggestions as to how to adapt these activities to the child who has visual and hearing impairments.

In Chapter 8 of Volume 1, we discussed the need for the individual with profound retardation to have an adequate cognitive basis in order to develop specific skills in other areas. Self-help skills, like communication skills, can only be acquired given sufficient prerequisite cognitive skills. For these reasons, initial programming in the self-help area of the curriculum may well involve targeting specified cognitive and motor prerequisites. The increasingly held view that skills should be taught within daily routines suggests that activities such as dressing and those involved at mealtimes offer extensive opportunities for targeting cognitive, motor and communication skills the development of which will in turn enable the individual to obtain a higher level of functioning in the self-help skills area. For example, McInnes and Treffry suggest that the activities associated with family routines provide an excellent basis for imitative and imaginative play.

This chapter will briefly review some of the work in the area of self-help skills that has taken place, focusing on toileting, dressing and feeding. Examples of the work on fire safety training which arises from the greater emphasis being placed on care in the community and has been reported more recently, will also be considered. Finally some general issues will be raised concerning the ways in which self-help skills are taught.

Toilet Training

More than any other area of self-help skills, toilet training is the one in which the consequences of *not* training are probably the most unacceptable to parents and professionals. Unlike mealtimes and dressing which can be limited to specific times of day, the consequences of a parent out in public with an adolescent or adult who is not trained cannot easily be hidden. A child or adult who is not toilet trained might be less attractive for the staff who work with them and may have their activities limited as the staffing ratio and resources required to deal with incontinence on outings or holidays is much greater. Furthermore, the health hazard created in institutions by having urine and faeces scattered about or worse still, smeared about by other residents, is clearly a major problem.

Reviews of research on behavioural approaches to toilet training are provided by Watson (1967) and Wehman (1979). Most of these studies involve the use of the techniques described in Chapter 2 of this volume, that is, task analysis, prompting and fading, imitation, shaping and rewarding. Simon (1981) describes recording when the person wets or soils for several days prior to starting training by checking them every half an hour. This technique, elsewhere referred to as the timing technique, can be very useful provided the intake of fluids occurs fairly consistently and at similar times each day. An example of this type of record is given in Figure 6.1.

Figure 6.1: Example of a Baseline Record Used in the Timing Technique for Toilet Training

	Monday				Tuesday				Wednesday			etc
	Dry	Wet	Soil		Dry	Wet	Soil		Dry	Wet	Soil	
7.30												
8.00												
8.30												
9.00												
9.30												
10.00												
10.30												

Source: Adapted from Simon, G.B. (1981), *The Next Step on the Ladder,* British Institute of Mental Handicap, Kidderminster. Reproduced by kind permission of the publishers BIMH Publications.

Any consistency in the times of wetting or soiling are identified and the person is taken to the toilet or placed on the potty just prior to these times in the hope of 'catching' them. They are then rewarded if they use the toilet or potty. Wetness, soiling or nonperformance on the toilet or potty are all ignored and dry pants always rewarded. Daytime training is always targeted first and only when well established does nightime training begin.

Wehman describes the 'rapid toilet training' technique introduced by Azrin and Foxx (1974) in order to reduce training time to 4–5 days. This procedure involves artifically increasing the amount of liquid

consumed by the client to ensure frequent urination, positive reinfo
ment for appropriate use of toilet, 'time out' for accidents and mal
the child or adult clean it up themselves. The client is encourage
initiate the visits to the toilet and is reinforced for being dry. An electr
sensor is fitted into the pants to ensure that the client and staff
informed immediately at the start of urination.

Rapid toilet training provides an apparently reliable way of trair
people who are profoundly retarded in a very short time. This has
obvious advantage of being likely to lead to success before staff
up the procedure and of being relatively rewarding in a short ti
However, there is currently increasing concern about teaching pe
skills in as 'natural' a setting as possible, that is teaching within the cor
of their daily lives. On this criterion the procedure clearly fails in
it requires almost exclusively toilet training for the 4–5 day period
a denial of other activities.

Ethical issues are raised by the question of how far urination or bc
movements should be manipulated for the purposes of training. G
and Wolf (1966) used laxatives in their programmes as well as restr
ing jackets and tying people to toilets. These procedures are unli!
to be acceptable in the current climate in which concern has b
expressed about how far it is possible to establish that the consen
the client has been given. Furthermore, the argument used by War
in 1967, that is, that the consequences of behaviour (i.e. not being tc
trained) are far worse than the inhumanity involved in the trair
procedures, can only be accepted if we are certain we cannot teach pe
to use the toilet by other methods.

It is apparent that other factors raised by Watson are still of releva
in the 1980s. The outcome of toilet training programmes is influen
by how far the environment on offer maintains the appropriate behavic
If there are acceptable staffing ratios, no overcrowding, easy acces
toilets and plenty of them and privacy in toilets, it seems probable
residents are far more likely to use them. Shrubsole and Smith (19
compared residents during a period when their wards were being moc
nised and they were in a portakabin unit which was uncomfortable, ov
crowded and lacking in facilities, with what they were like when t
had settled back into their refurbished wards. The level of contine
significantly increased for the 13 adults with profound retardation v
were studied in the refurbished ward conditions. The authors conclu
that overcrowding, boredom and poor amenities influence both the le
of incontinence and the success of training programmes. Further evide
of the effects of overcrowding comes from Hereford, Cleland and Fell

(1973) who found that increasing the available territory led to a decrease in nocturnal wetting and soiling in males with profound retardation.

The issue raised by Watson regarding the need for staff to receive encouragement, in order to maintain programmes, has often been stated in the literature over the past 20 years not only in relation to programmes on toilet training. However, maintaining a consistent approach between all people coming into contact with the client remains one of the most insoluble problems since there is always the possibility of one person, whether bus driver or supply teacher, unaware of the programme, responding differently. To reiterate the point made in Chapter 2, programmes in which the main procedures are summarised in written form and are kept readily available may minimise this problem.

Many intriguing devices have been introduced in toilet training. Watson described the use of automated reinforcer dispensers and flashing lights and proposed the possible use of electronically bugged pants which have since become fairly common. Jones (1983), for example, describes in detail (including diagrams) how to devise such pants, electronic bed sensors and fitted sensors in toilets. At the Anson House project (Gunstone, Hogg, Sebba, Warner and Almond 1982) musical potties were used with some success. All of this equipment provides more economical and reliable methods of toilet training as it depends less on staff to dispense rewards. It also enables immediate rewards to be given without interrupting the client every few moments to inspect the contents of the potty or toilet in order to decide whether a reward is due. Levitt (1982) provides useful examples of ways in which children with physical impairments can be assisted to maintain postural stability through the use of rails for them to grasp.

Further guidelines and examples of toilet training programmes for people with profound and multiple impairments can be found in Wehman (1979), Jegard, Anderson, Glazer and Zaleski (1980), Simon (1981) and McInnes and Treffry (1982). McInnes and Treffry provide specific suggestions for the client with hearing and visual impairments. They advocate the use of the co-active approach described fully in Chapter 2 of this volume for all self-help skills including toileting. The child with sensory impairments should be manipulated co-actively through the processes for a considerable length of time, before any attempt is made to actually teach the skills involved. The emphasis during the first stage is to give the child the same degree of awareness and understanding of what is happening as that acquired by the nonhandicapped child through the use of sight and hearing. McInnes and Treffry point out that since most of our 'grooming' checks are visual, alternative methods of checking will need to be developed, for example, learning to recognise the feel of a skirt caught up by tights after using the toilet. Jegard *et al.* and Simon provide specific suggestions for those with physical impairments, in addition to suggestions for coping with sensory impairments.

Dressing

Dressing, like toilet training, has been taught more commonly by the use of the techniques described in Chapter 2 of this volume, that is task analysis, shaping, prompting, fading and rewarding. An early study by Minge and Ball (1967) showed that by using a programmed learning approach consisting of task analysis to determine small enough steps and with appropriate reinforcement six people with profound retardation were taught dressing and undressing skills. The skills were taught in their natural context, in this case at shower time and bedtime. It was noted that the people trained were more attentive and showed less unacceptable behaviours after the skills had been established. This was one of the earliest studies to demonstrate that undressing skills were more readily acquired than dressing skills. However, a later study by Ball, Seric and Payne (1971) noted that although undressing skills were learnt more quickly by children with profound retardation they were not maintained, whereas dressing skills were acquired over years. The researchers concluded that this was due to the nonverbal cues in the ward situation that occur naturally everyday to prompt dressing, such as silently handing out T-shirts to be put on. Undressing on the other hand requires more structured verbal instructions and physical prompts which are less likely to occur naturally in an institution.

The importance of considering long-term maintenance of skills was not taken into account in the study of 'rapid' dressing training (Azrin, Schaeffer and Wesolowski 1976) involving a similar approach to the rapid toilet training procedure, in order to achieve mastery of skills in a minimal time period. Seven adults with profound retardation (but without physical impairments) were taught to dress and undress totally independently within 20 hours of training over 4 days. The average time taken to master the skills to criterion was 2 days of 5 hours' training per day. The procedure involved teaching undressing first with a major emphasis on physical prompting and fading, continuous instructions throughout the task and using reinforcers intrinsic to the task, for example by showing them in a mirror at each stage as well as continuous praise and stroking. Initially, larger sizes of clothing were used and the person was trained on the entire sequence, that is, forward chaining using all the articles to be taken off. This was an unusual aspect of the procedure as most training manuals (e.g. Wehman 1979 and Simon 1981) suggest using backward chaining for the steps in dressing or undressing tasks and concentrating on one item of clothing at a time.

The rapid dressing procedure has similar shortcomings to those discussed in relation to rapid toilet training. The intensity of the training necessitates teaching the skills outside of the natural opportunities to dress and undress that occur during daily routines and must be at the expense of most other activities. Furthermore, a recent attempt (Diorio and Konarski 1984) to replicate the Azrin *et al.* study with three adults with profound retardation, could not reach criterion of dressing skills with any of the clients and one failed to reach criterion on the undressing skills. The procedure was still regarded as successful as important skills were gained, although not to a level of complete independence, and generalisation occurred across trainers, in that it was demonstrated that direct care staff as well as psychologists could act as successful trainers. No support was noted for the Ball *et al.* contention that dressing skills were maintained over the long term, since follow-ups at 1, 2, 3 and 10 months indicated that skills were only maintained up to 3 months.

Similar techniques to those described above have been used to teach students with multiple impairments to put on their hearing aids (Tucker and Berry 1980). Although not an activity usually termed 'dressing', it would seem appropriate to include it here since it might be assumed that the aid is put on and taken off whenever clothes are put on and taken off. Task analysis was used to identify 10 steps in this procedure and each student was taught selective steps according to their individual needs for training, which were determined partly by their motor skills and the type of aid worn. All six students trained achieved criterion but the one student who was profoundly retarded showed more variability in the accuracy of his performance. Four of the six, including the one with profound retardation, spontaneously generalised their newly acquired skills to both classroom and residential unit.

Some of the clearest examples of instructional packages on dressing are those developed by Hofmeister and Reavis (1974), examples of which are also given in Atkinson (1977). These are clearly illustrated and very basic training procedures for instructional aides and parents. They are derived from the theory of direct instruction (Engelmann and Carnine 1982) which is applied through a model, lead, test, review procedure. The skill is modelled by the trainer, who then leads the client through it (e.g. 'Let's do it together') and finally tests the client on the skill by asking them to do it on their own. The whole procedure is reviewed to ensure the skills have been mastered. Scripted formats are given, suggesting exactly what the person should do at each stage when teaching an unmastered skill or concept to a learner who is severely or profoundly intellectually impaired. Each unit covering a skill or set of skills lists the prerequisite skills required by the learner. Correction procedures and techniques for practising the new skill are also given. The packages include suggestions for reinforcement procedures, pre/post unit criterion-referenced tests and procedures for continuous monitoring of progress. They have been fully evaluated. The only disadvantage with these packages appear to be their suggested use of token economy systems of reinforcement, the use of which, as we discussed in Chapter 2, is limited with those whose cognitive disabilities are most profound.

An example of part of the programme on teaching the independent use of zippers, buttons, shoes and socks is given in Figure 6.2.

Levitt (1982) provides a developmental sequence for dressing skills with practical suggestions for teaching them to children with physical impairments. She notes that the contexts of dressing activities can provide additional opportunities to develop perception, balance, movements and communication. McInnes and Treffry (1982) describe examples of how the child who has sensory impairments can be manipulated co-actively through dressing activities, each activity being extended to create an awareness of the next stage. For example, undressing activities can be extended to include awareness of putting the dirty clothes in a wash basket by co-actively following procedures which do this. These authors also provide suggestions for building in maintenance and generalisation activities, for example, by creating circumstances in which the child puts on his or her sweater inside out, in order to provide the opportunity to teach recognition of this situation and how it can be remedied.

Suggestions are given by Levitt of ways in which clothes can be adapted to make dressing easier for people with physical impairments, for example, by using Velcro and zips rather than laces and smaller fastenings. We have stressed the importance of teaching skills within the context in which they are needed and for this reason, find the use of 'models' or 'dummies' less acceptable. The child, as McInnes and Treffry point out, could learn to lace and tie shoes on the dummy but the procedure would be the opposite of that actually needed, since the 'dummy's' right would be the child's left and vice versa.

Other useful examples of dressing programmes can be found in Wehman (1979), Jegard *et al.* (1980) and Simon (1981). Wehman provides a teaching objective analysed into 30 steps for putting on and

Figure 6.2: Part of a Programme on Teaching the Independent Use of Zippers and Buttons.

I: (Rezip the jacket.)

Now, let's do it together. I will help. First, we hold the tab with this hand.

(Help the learner hold the tab with the thumb and forefinger of one hand.)

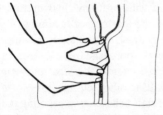

L: (Holds the zipper tab with instructor's help.)

> **TO CORRECT:** Remember *tell, show, help, praise.* If the learner has trouble, *tell* him how to do it. If he still has trouble, *show* him how to do it. If he still has trouble, *help* him do it. *Praise* him when he does it by himself.

I: Now, we slide the zipper tab down to the bottom.

(Slide the zipper tab to the bottom, *but not off* the track.)

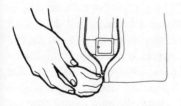

L: (Slides zipper down, *but not off* the track, with the instructor's help.)

I: That's the way to slide the tab! Next, we hold the side of the zipper with this hand.

(Help the learner hold the side of the zipper with the thumb and forefinger.)

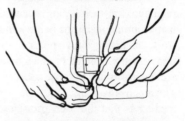

L: (Holds the side of the zipper with the instructor's help.)

I: Now, we hold and pull *up* on this side of the zipper while pulling *down* on the tab.

(Help the learner unzip his jacket.)

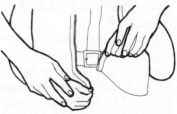

L: (Unzips his jacket with the instructor's help.)

I: There, we did it! We unzipped the jacket.

(Repeat Step B until the learner correctly completes each part of the step with your help. When he does, proceed to Step C.)

Source: Atkinson, C.M. (1977, p. 9), 'Programming for the Untrained Instructional Aide' in J. Cronin (ed.), *The Severely and Profoundly Handicapped Child,* State Board of Education, Illinois.

fastening lace-up shoes and one with 53 steps for putting on and fastening a pair of trousers.

Feeding

The importance of establishing good drinking and feeding patterns is stressed by Warner (1981) and Levitt (1982) who both point out that development of the oral musculature that occurs in feeding is a prerequisite for developing speech. Self-feeding and the reduction of inappropriate mealtime behaviours have provided the main focus for the work on eating skills relating to people with profound and multiple impairments. The techniques involved in the teaching of feeding skills are again similar to those used in teaching dressing and toilet training. The main advantage with the behavioural approaches in the area of feeding is that the food provides, for most clients, the ideal intrinsic reward. The issues of generalisation of skills to other settings, long-term maintenance of skills and maintenance of staff behaviour in carrying out programmes are central to all areas of self-help skill training. Typically, the studies reported involve small numbers of people with profound retardation, usually in an institution, being taught to feed themselves with spoons.

One example of this type of study (Song and Gandhi 1974) involved using a seven-step shaping procedure to teach self-feeding in which it was noted that scooping the food was by far the most difficult step. Although no systematic maintenance procedure was required, the trainers needed feedback to ensure continuation of the programmes. Another study (McDonald, McCabe and Mackle 1977) did not find that the trained skills were maintained once training had ceased, but the peripheral skills, such as carrying the food to the table and clearing away the plates at the end of the meal, increased and remained increased even when training on the spoon feeding had ended. The authors postulated that this was due to poor staff ratios on the ward which led to staff feeding clients to save time whereas the peripheral skills contributed to the ward routine however slowly they were done.

The issue of how far staff assist residents in skills they are able to carry out independently, if left to do so, has been taken up more recently by Cullen (1986). Cullen refers to the Offerton Self-Care Checklist (Burton, Thomas and Cullen 1981) which provides a criterion-referenced assessment of self-care skills starting with a checklist on staff behaviour to establish whether residents are given the opportunity to carry out their own self-care skills. It is not only staff interaction with residents in terms of assistance given that is of interest, but also aspects of the environment such as the ward routine which may contribute to whether residents have the chance to serve themselves to food, collect their utensils and so on.

An attempt to create 'normalised' mealtimes for people with profound retardation and to observe the effects is reported by Wilson, Reid, Phillips and Burgio (1984). All four residents could eat with a spoon and fork with staff supervision but were trained on 12 steps of premeal skills (e.g. fetching plate), 9 steps of mealtime behaviour (e.g. serving food) and 9 steps of post-meal skills (e.g. clearing table). All showed total or near-total independence in preparing, eating and clearing up with their peers after training. This was generalised to all their meals and maintained throughout follow-up, but unlike McDonald *et al.*'s study, Wilson *et al.* noted that peripheral skills observed such as peer communication and improved mealtime neatness (e.g. not eating directly from the serving dish) did not improve. These authors concluded that caution is therefore needed in assuming that creating normalised mealtimes will necessarily have multiple benefits in relation to specific skills, each skill requiring direct training.

Another study noting generalisation of training effects to other self-help skills is that reported by Kissel, Whitman and Reid (1983). They found that when direct care staff were trained to carry out behavioural techniques to teach toothbrushing to residents with profound retardation, improvement occurred not only on toothbrushing skills but also on hair-combing and handwashing skills. The question of whether each skill requires direct training therefore remains unclear.

It will be of no surprise that Azrin and Armstrong (1973) suggested a method of rapidly training eating skills to persons with profound retardation. The 'mini-meal' method involves dividing the regular meals up into smaller portions given hourly to allow for more sessions and minimise satiation. Similar techniques were used as in the rapid toilet training and dressing programmes except that distractions were minimised by limiting the utensils and giving no verbal prompts. All eleven residents learned to eat independently in an average of 5 training days compared to only 4 out of the 11 residents in an 'intensive programme' control group. The skills had been maintained 7 months after training on follow-up.

The mini-meal has the same problems as the other rapid training techniques. It distorts the daily lives of the clients and staff and would seem in sharp contrast to the attempt reported above to create 'normalised mealtimes' for people with profound retardation. The rapid training methods are apparently successful in establishing skills and seem to be used by the relatively few staff who are committed to them.

There are many behaviour problems associated with eating behaviour and although behaviour problems are discussed fully in the next chapter, it may be worth considering how studies of these help to identify the positive aspects of teaching feeding skills. Many examples can be found of programmes designed to teach self-feeding resulting in a reduction of inappropriate mealtime behaviour. Sixty residents with severe and profound retardation were reported by Groves and Carroccio (1971) to be trained to use a spoon appropriately with a reduction of food stealing and hand feeding. Likewise, Albin (1977) found that teaching three children with profound retardation to spoon feed reduced finger feeding and stealing food. These studies are supporting the approach to dealing with behaviour problems, known as differential reinforcement of incompatible behaviour (DRI), reviewed in the next chapter, since both food stealing and hand feeding cannot be carried out if the person's hands are busy spoon feeding themselves.

Another general issue raised in the next chapter but mentioned by Albin in relation to the feeding programme described is the lack of maintenance of appropriate eating behaviour which occurs in some residential settings in which these people live. For example, if the child attempts to communicate nonverbally that he or she would like a second helping and this attempt is ignored or misunderstood the child may learn to steal the food. Another example would be in situations in which the individual has received a plate of food but no utensils with which to eat it, so the person uses his or her fingers. Kiernan and Reid (1986) have suggested that this type of manipulation of the routine might assist in the facilitation of communication by giving the individual a reason to communicate. Hence, we must carefully weigh up each situation in order to provide maximum opportunities to communicate by not letting routines run too smoothly, without allowing the situation to be used by the client to develop a behaviour problem.

Other attempts to reduce inappropriate mealtime behaviour have used facial disapproval, verbal castigation and physical restraint (Henriksen 1967) and time out in the form of removing the tray of food (Christian, Holloman and Lanier 1973) amongst other approaches. A particular problem in the area of feeding concerns chronic regurgitation and self-vomiting. Ball, Hendricksen and Clayton (1974) used special feeding methods including stimulation in different areas of the mouth with a spoon and streams of milk and active participation in the feeding process by the child to reduce voluntary regurgitation. A study carried out by one of the current authors (Hogg 1982) and described more fully in the next chapter, demonstrated the effectiveness of lemon juice to reduce self-induced vomiting in a child with multiple impairments. Finally a problem not limited to populations with mental retardation, that of anorexia, which Carson and Morgan (1974) successfully treated in a girl with profound mental retardation by using a secondary reinforcer (in this case, a bell) to re-establish a primary reinforcer, the food.

Guidelines on teaching feeding skills are provided in Jegard *et al.* (1980), Wehman (1979), Simon (1981), Levitt (1982) and McInnes and Treffry (1982). Levitt produces a developmental sequence of feeding skills with practical suggestions for teaching, stressing, as do McInnes and Treffry, the importance of remaining unhurried and of ensuring the child is in a good position, when feeding. Both these texts describe methods of weaning from liquidised food to semi-solid and solid food and Levitt describes methods of coping with gagging, chocking and drooling. Both emphasise the procedural adaptations that can be used to assist people who have sensory and physical impairments.

The checklist and manual produced by Warner (1981) on early feeding skills also provides clear and useful guidelines with excellent illustrations. Jegard *et al.*, Simon, Warner and Wehman also go into detail on issues such as when to feed the child, positioning, swallowing, straw drinking, using a cup, chewing and feeding with a spoon. Examples of guidelines from Simon, Warner and Wehman are given in Figures 6.3, 6.4 and 6.5.

Many of these skills are now being taught in conjunction with advice from speech therapists. The relationship between the establishment of appropriate feeding and drinking patterns and early speech was mentioned at the start of this chapter and in Chapter 4 of this volume. Intervention with people with profound and multiple impairments in order to establish these patterns has therefore become of interest to teacher and speech therapist alike.

Special Equipment. Many of the texts mentioned above include suggestions for special feeding and drinking equipment which assist people with multiple impairments. Watson (1967) and Wehman (1979) mention spoons with build up handles, partitioned tables which keep children's food separate, plates with high sides, sloping cups with lids with spouts, etc. More suggestions are given in Ryan (1976), Simon (1981), Warner (1981) and Levitt (1982). Levitt suggests that the occupational therapist should be consulted, where possible, about the correct selection of feeding aids in each individual case.

Figure 6.3: Example of Guidelines on Finger Feeding

You may feel that it is unnecessary to teach the child to eat with his fingers and would prefer to go straight on to spoon feeding. However, finger feeding will encourage him to accept food, such as a biscuit, when offered by hand and it will help him learn to control the use of his hands and fingers.

When the child is eating and chewing on a variety of solids, teach him to feed himself with his fingers from a bowl and plate. Always put him in the *same* place for his food, preferably sitting at a low table, with his feet on the floor or on the foot rest of his chair.

Always put his food into a heavy bowl or plate on a non-slip surface. A rubber pad placed underneath the bowl will prevent it from slipping and can be purchased at most chemists' shops. In the early stages it will help him if you put his plate in the same place in front of him each time.

To begin with, guide the child's hands into the bowl and get him to pick up a piece of food, then guide his hand to his mouth. Let go when he can chew on it, as he has already learned this. When he has finished that piece of food, guide his hand back to the bowl for a second piece.

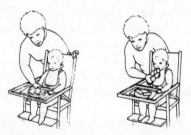

Finger feeding helps the child learn to control the use of his hands as well as encouraging him to hold foods such as sandwiches and biscuits.

You may find that the child will not eat much himself at first but if, at every meal-time, you get him used to the same procedure he will learn where his food is, how to reach it and how to get it into his mouth. As he progresses you can begin to let go of his hand a little further away from his mouth so that gradually he has to complete more and more of the whole action himself. Continue this until you are giving him only minimal assistance, perhaps just touching his hand to show him the right movement.

Source: Simon, G.B. (1981, p. 89), *The Next Step on the Ladder,* British Institute of Mental Handicap, Kidderminster. Reproduced by kind permission of the publishers BIMH Publications.

Figure 6.4: Example of Guidelines on Lip Control

The aim of these exercises is to encourage lip closure.

Put your finger between the nose and the upper lip, stroke down several times and then put your finger under the lower lip and push up. Sometimes pressing the lower lip down for a short time will help the lip spring back.

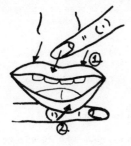
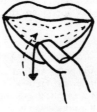

If the upper lip is pulled back in a grimace, run your fingers down the side of the nose to the corners of the mouth. Pushing the upper lip up a little at first may help.

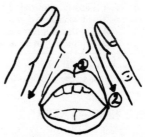

Using two fingers press the upper and lower lips together. Try to make lip smacking sounds to ensure a firm closure.

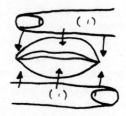

Source: Warner (1981 p. 42).

Figure 6.5: Example of Guidelines on Swallowing

Swallowing

To teach voluntary swallowing, the following steps should be followed:
1. The head should be in a slightly downward position.
2. Use only a small amount of liquid in the cup; it is easier and keeps the child from being discouraged.
3. Stroke the throat to facilitate swallowing.
4. Discourage the child from biting the cup.
5. If there is no lip closure (due to overbite or involuntary motion), hold the lips shut with very slight finger pressure to the upper and lower lips.
6. Teach the child to take one sip and swallow.
7. If the child stiffens as the cup approaches, wait until he relaxes again. He will soon learn that he will get food only when relaxed.

Straw-Drinking

Straw drinking can be started whether the hands are ready or not. There are several important factors to remember:
1. It is a step towards independent feeding.
2. It is a prespeech activity (breath control for example).
3. It helps in controlling drooling.
4. It is an excellent means of getting liquids into a severely involved child.
    A. Use a short plastic straw with a small circumference.
    B. Only a small amount of liquid should be placed in the cup.

Source: Wehman (1979, p. 40), *Curriculum Design for the Severely and Profoundly Handicapped,* Human Sciences Press, New York

Other Self-help Skills

According to the definition accepted of self-help skills, a whole range of additional skills could be covered here including shopping, cooking, cleaning and so on. Perhaps, if one considers the skills most likely to be taught to people with profound mental retardation, then they have probably been covered by those described above. However, recent plans for closure of hospitals and expansions in residential provision in the community has meant that even those people whose level of retardation is most profound are sometimes considered for community placement. In the USA, one of the criteria which can determine whether community placement is possible is the speed with which the resident can evacuate the building on hearing a fire alarm. The State Laws specify the time within which the residents must be able to leave the building.

In response to these requirements Cohen (1984) reports training, in 2.5 hours, a blind 30 year old man with profound retardation to exit independently from a community residence within 28.5 seconds. Cohen used a forward chaining procedure involving 10 steps and quotes evidence suggesting that this behaviour does not correlate with the level of cognitive functioning. Rae and Roll (1985) used a once a day training programme (varying times of the day) to teach 10 adults with profound retardation one of whom was blind and another epileptic to evacuate the building faster. The average time taken was reduced from 87 seconds to 24 seconds over a year of daily training and was upheld for 4 months with weekly fire drills only.

This work on responding appropriately in situations of potential danger would seem to fall naturally into the self-help area of the curriculum. It is apparent that the increase in possibilities for people with profound and multiple impairments to reside in the community will demand further training in health and safety skills. Jarman, Iwata and Lorentzson (1983) have argued that teaching sequences of self-help skills will also become increasingly important as these skills rarely occur in isolation (e.g. washing and feeding, toileting and washing, etc.). Independent living will require people to be able to sequence these skills in the appropriate order at the appropriate time.

Further consideration will need to be given to whether self-help skills training should occur on an individual basis or in groups. If we apply the principles of normalisation to this question then perhaps the training should be individualised when we want the behaviour to be individual as for example in toileting. There is no longer any justification for conducting toilet training in groups if the people concerned are accepted as having individualised toileting needs and are to be expected to use individual public toilets. On the other hand, mealtimes for most of this population will always be a group activity. Hence, mealtime behaviour could be trained in groups, with individualised targets to remove the necessity for the behaviour to generalise to a group setting. It is clear that however the training is conducted, consideration will still need to be given to ensuring that the environment in which people live maximises their opportunities for practising self-help skills independently.

References

Albin, J.B. (1977) 'Some Variables Influencing the Maintenance of Acquired Self-Feeding Behavior in Profoundly Retarded Children', *Mental Retardation, 15*, 49–52

Atkinson, C.M. (1977) 'Programming for the Untrained Instructional Aide' in

J. Cronin (ed.), *The Severely and Profoundly Handicapped Child*, State Board of Education, Illinois

Azrin, N.H. and Armstrong, P.M. (1973) 'The Mini-Meal — A Method for Teaching Eating Skills to the Profoundly Retarded, *Mental Retardation, 11*, 9–13

Azrin, N.H. and Foxx, R.M. (1974) *Toilet Training in Less than a Day*, Simon and Schuster, New York

Azrin, N.H., Schaeffer, R.M. and Wesolowski, M.D. (1976) 'A Rapid Method of Teaching Profoundly Retarded Persons to Dress by a Reinforcement-Guidance Method', *Mental Retardation, 14*, 29–33

Ball, T.S., Hendricksen, H. and Clayton, J. (1974) 'A Special Feeding Technique for Chronic Regurgitation', *American Journal of Mental Deficiency, 78*, 486–93

Ball, T.S., Seric, K. and Payne, L.E. (1971) 'Long-term Retention of Self-help Skill Training in the Profoundly Retarded', *American Journal of Mental Deficiency, 76*, 378–82

Balthazar, E.E., Naor, E.M. and Sindberg, R.M. (1973) 'Absence of Intervention Training Programmes: Effects Upon the Severely and Profoundly Retarded' in Central Winsconsin Colony and Training School Research Department (eds.), *Monograph Supplement Number 1*

Bensberg, G.J., Colwell, C.N. and Cassell, R.H. (1965) 'Teaching the Profoundly Retarded Self-Help Activities by Behavior-Shaping Techniques', *American Journal of Mental Deficiency, 69*, 674–9

Burton, M., Thomas, M. and Cullen, C. (1981) 'Offerton Self-Care Checklist', unpublished manuscript, Hester Adrian Research Centre, University of Manchester, Manchester

Carson, P. and Morgan, S.B. (1974) 'Behavior Modification of Food Aversion in a Profoundly Retarded Female: A Case Study', *Psychological Reports, 34*, 954

Christian, W.P., Holloman, S.W. and Lanier, C.L. (1973) 'An Attendant Operated Feeding Program for Severely and Profoundly Retarded Females', *Mental Retardation, 11*, 35–7

Cohen, I.L. (1984) 'Establishment of Independent Responding to a Fire Alarm in a Blind, Profoundly Retarded Adult', *Journal of Behavior Therapy and Experimental Psychiatry, 15*, 365–7

Cullen, C. (1986) 'Nurse Training and Insititutional Constraints' in J. Hogg and P. Mittler (eds.), *Staff Training in Mental Handicap*, Croom Helm, London

Diorio, M.S. and Konarski, E.A. (1984) 'Evaluation of a Method for Teaching Dressing Skills to Profoundly Mentally Retarded Persons', *American Journal of Mental Deficiency, 89*, 307–9

Engelmann, S. and Carnine, D. (1982) *Theory of Instruction: Principles and Applications*, Irvington, New York

Giles, D.K. and Wolf, M.M. (1966) 'Toilet Training Institutionalised, Severe Retardates: An Application of Operant Behavior Modification Techniques', *American Journal of Mental Deficiency, 70*, 766–80

Groves, I.D. and Carroccio, D.E. (1971) 'A Self-Feeding Program for the Severely and Profoundly Retarded', *Mental Retardation, 9*, 10–12

Gunstone, C., Hogg, J., Sebba, J., Warner, J. and Almond, S. (1982) *Classroom Provision and Organisation for Integrated Preschool Children*, Barnardo's

Publications, Barkingside

Henriksen, K. (1967) 'Decelerating Undesired Mealtime Behavior in a Group of Profoundly Retarded Boys', *American Journal of Mental Deficiency, 72,* 40–4

Hereford, S.M., Cleland, C.C. and Fellner, M. (1973) 'Territoriality and Scent Making: A Study of Profoundly Retarded Enuretics and Encopretics', *American Journal of Mental Deficiency, 77,* 426–30

Hofmeister, A.M. and Reavis, H.K. (1974) 'Packages for Parent Involvement', *Educational Technology, 14,* 55–6

Hogg, J. (1982) 'Reduction of Self-Induced Vomiting in a Multiply Handicapped Girl by "Lemon Juice Therapy" and Concomitant Changes in Social Behaviour', *British Journal of Clinical Psychology, 21,* 227–8

Jarman, P.H., Iwata, B.A. and Lorentzson, A.M. (1983) 'Development of Morning Self-Care Routines in Multiply Handicapped Persons', *Applied Research in Mental Retardation, 4,* 113–22

Jegard, S., Anderson, L., Glazer, C. and Zaleski, W.A. (1980) *A Comprehensive Program for Multihandicapped Children: An Illustrated Approach,* Alvin Buckwold Centre, Saskatchewan

Jones, M. (1983) *Behaviour Problems in Handicapped Children,* Souvenir Press, London

Kiernan, C.C. and Reid, B. (1986) *Pre-Verbal Communication Schedule (PVC) Manual,* NFER-Nelson, Windsor

Kissel, R.C., Whitman, T.L. and Reid, D.H. (1983) 'An Institutional Staff Training and Self Management Program for Developing Multiple Self-Care Skills in Severely/Profoundly Retarded Individuals', *Journal of Applied Behavior Analysis, 16,* 395–415

Levitt, S. (1982) *Treatment of Cerebral Palsy and Motor Delay,* Blackwell, Oxford

McDonald, G., McCabe, P. and Mackle, B. (1977) 'Mealtime Behaviour in the Profoundly Subnormal', *British Journal of Mental Subnormality, 23,* 29–35

McInnes, J.M. and Treffry, J.A. (1982) *Deaf-Blind Infants and Children: A Development Guide,* University of Toronto Press, Toronto/Open University Press, Milton Keynes

Minge, R.M. and Ball, T.S. (1967) 'Teaching of Self-Help Skills to Profoundly Retarded Patients', *American Journal of Mental Deficiency, 71,* 864–8

Rae, R. and Roll, D. (1985) 'Fire Safety Training with Adults who are Profoundly Mentally Retarded', *Mental Retardation, 23,* 26–30

Ryan, M. (1976) *Feeding Can Be Fun: Advice on Feeding Handicapped Babies and Children,* Spastics Society, London

Shrubsole, L. and Smith, P.S. (1984) 'The Effects of Change of Environment on Daytime Incontinence in Profoundly Mentally Handicapped Adults', *British Journal of Mental Subnormality, 30,* 44–53

Simon, G.B. (1981) *The Next Step on the Ladder,* British Institute of Mental Handicap, Kidderminster

Song, A.Y. and Gandhi, R. (1974) 'An Analysis of Behavior During the Acquisition and Maintenance Phases of Self-Spoon Feeding Skills of Profound Retardates', *Mental Retardation, 12,* 25–8

Tucker, D.J. and Berry, G.W. (1980) 'Teaching Severely Multihandicapped Students to put on their own Hearing Aids', *Journal of Applied Behavior*

Analysis, 13, 65–75

Warner, J. (1981) *Helping the Handicapped Child with Early Feeding,* Winslow Press, Buckingham

Watson, L.S. (1967) 'Application of Operant Conditioning Techniques to Institutionalised Severely and Profoundly Retarded Children', *Mental Retardation Abstracts, 4,* 1–18

Wehman, P. (1979) *Curriculum Design for the Severely and Profoundly Handicapped,* Human Sciences Press, New York

Wilson, P.G., Reid, D.H., Phillips, J.F. and Burgio, L.D. (1984) 'Normalisation of Institutional Mealtimes of Profoundly Retarded Persons: Effects and Non-Effects of Teaching Family-Style Dining', *Journal of Applied Behavior Analysis, 17,* 189–201

7 BEHAVIOUR PROBLEMS

Introduction

In Chapter 1 of the first volume of this book, we drew attention to two aspects of behaviour problems in relation to profound retardation and multiple impairments. First, we pointed out that, contrary to some definitions of profound retardation and multipie impairment, we did not regard the presence of a behaviour problem as one of the criteria by which a person should be considered profoundly retarded and multiply impaired. Put in another way, the presence of a behaviour problem was not considered as an 'additional impairment' in the same sense in which physical or sensory impairments are so regarded. Second, we noted that there is no simple definition of what constitutes a behaviour problem and hence no assessment instrument that can be used to ascertain objectively the presence of such a problem. (For a full discussion of problems of definition in relation to available assessment procedures see Leudar and Fraser 1986).

Both the problems of definition and those of assessment led us to conclude that it is difficult if not impossible to establish the exact proportion of people who are profoundly retarded and multiply impaired *and* who exhibit behaviour problems. Nevertheless, it was pointed out that there is a strong suggestion in the literature that as we move through increasing degress of retardation, so the presence of such problems increases. If this picture is somewhat inexact, there can be little doubt that anyone working with children or adults in the group with whom we are concerned will have to deal with many individuals whose behaviour presents problems for themselves or others.

This chapter is concerned with approaches to intervention aimed at preventing or eliminating behaviour problems. In order to consider such intervention, however, some preliminary account of behaviour disorders should be given. First, what is the range of such disorders and how might we group them for purposes of discussion? Secondly, what do we know about the origins of various types of behaviour disorders and, thirdly, what does this suggest regarding general teaching strategies? Finally, we then offer some illustrations in a little more detail of programmes that have been undertaken with some representative behaviour problems.

Types of Behaviour Problems

A thorough description of types of behaviour problems has come from the work of Nihira (1978) using Part II of the Adaptive Behavior Scale (Nihira, Foster, Shellhaas and Leland 1974). This scale presents a wide range of behaviour problems that have been reported by staff in schools, training centres and institutions working with people who are mentally handicapped. A 'problem' here is defined in terms of what is seen to be a problem by staff when working in a particular setting with a given individual. A range of general classes of behaviour can be scored on the scale, e.g. whether the person does or does not threaten or show aggressive behaviour to others, followed by recording specific instances of such behaviour, e.g that the client bites others.

Nihira (1978) had staff in a number of institutions rate their residents on all scales. Of special interest here is the fact that he grouped those rated not only in terms of age (10–18 years vs 19–69), but also into mildly/moderately retarded vs severe/profound, though more detailed information on profound retardation alone is not given. However, the distinction between these ability groupings was not great with respect to the various types of behaviour problems, i.e. with a few exceptions the severe/profound groups showed the same type of problems in similar measure. Three general categories of behaviour were regarded as reflecting social maladaptation and three categories as reflecting personal maladaptation. These are listed below with specific examples of the kinds of behaviour typifying them:

SOCIAL MALADAPTATION
  1 *Violent and antisocial behaviour*
          — threatens or does physical violence
          — has violent temper or tantrums
          — teases or gossips about others
          — bosses and manipulates others
          — uses angry language
          — reacts poorly to criticism or frustration
  2 *Rebellious behaviour*
          — ignores regulations and routines
          — resists following directions
          — is impudent or rebellious
          — absents self from places at times arranged
          — runs away
          — misbehaves in group settings

3 *Untrustworthy behaviour*
- shows disrespect for other's property
- runs away
- takes other's property without permission
- lies or cheats

PERSONAL MALADAPTATION

4 *Destructive behaviour towards property or self*
- damages personal property
- damages other's personal property
- damages public property
- disrupts others activities
- does physical violence to self

5 *Stereotyped and hyperactive behaviour*
- has stereotyped behaviours
- has inappropriate interpersonal manners
- has disturbing vocal or speech habits
- has hyperactive tendencies
- demands excessive attention or praise

6 *Inappropriate body exposure*
- removes or tears off own clothing
- engages in inappropriate masturbation
- exposes body improperly

While the categories of behaviour under Social Maladaptation are seen in both groups, i.e. mild/moderate and severe/profound, we would expect them to be more prevalent in the former (mild/moderate) group. Indeed, some of the concepts, such as lying or cheating, can have little meaning in the case of profound retardation when we consider the associated developmental level. Nihira does point out that behaviours in categories 2 and 3, i.e. rebellious and untrustworthy behaviour, are more frequent in the mild/moderate group. Conversely, many of the behaviours in the Personal Maladaptation categories will be seen in individuals who are profoundly retarded, i.e. self-injurious or stereotyped behaviour. For some individuals in this group, severe motor impairments will, however, preclude such behaviour developing. Eyman and Call (1977) report that where the physical capacity exists, people who are profoundly retarded are more likely to display self-injurious behaviour than those who are more able.

The issue of frequency, or the relation between ability and type of behaviour problem, is not what concerns us here. Nihira's study suggests that the framework of Social vs Personal Maladaptation is a useful one from which to select areas of behaviour problems in the group with which we are concerned both with respect to intervention and to their causes, to which we now turn.

The Origins of Behaviour Problems

In Volume 1, Chapter 3 we described a view of human development that sees behaviour as emerging from an interaction between the maturing child and his or her environment. This view has been called 'the ecological perspective on development'. It acknowledges that while the child brings a repertoire of behaviour to any situation, the way in which the environment responds will have a profound bearing, for good or ill, on future development. Where some impairment exists, then normally occurring patterns of interaction may be distorted, leading to different patterns of development from those expected for the nonimpaired child. In Chapter 4 of that volume, we described how visual impairment affected development in children who were otherwise unimpaired, noting how visual impairment could lead to behaviour disorders. Specifically, we reviewed evidence showing an association between visual impairment and behaviours such as stereotyped hand movements (often in front of the face) and body rocking. We also reviewed evidence that such behaviours may not result from visual deprivation alone, but deprivation to sensory input to the body resulting from reduced mobility. The nature of the interaction between the person and the environment was emphasised by the suggestion of one author that deprivation of this sort could lead to changes in brain functioning.

Similarly, in Volume 1, Chapter 5 we described the development of behaviour disorders in hearing impaired children. Here the main conclusion drawn was that the '. . . absence of communication in the global sense leads to behaviour problems . . .' (Schlesinger and Meadow 1972 p. 121), though the development of resulting behaviour problems has received little study. It was also pointed out that, where deafness was part of a wider pattern of multiple handicap, then the likelihood of behaviour disorders increased, depending on the site of any brain damage.

Behaviour disorders resulting from physical impairments were considered in Volume 1, Chapter 6. Again, an association between physical impairment or physical isolation and the emergence of behaviour disorders was documented.

In the three areas reviewed, therefore, we see that even in the absence of mental retardation in the conventional sense, highly specific sensory and physical impairments lead to a distortion in the person's interaction with the world resulting in behaviour problems. Where extensive brain damage exists, this course of events may be even more severely detrimental.

In Chapter 8 of Volume 1 we related the above findings to the development of behaviour problems in individuals who are profoundly retarded and multiply impaired. We suggested that while the ecological model is as appropriate to an understanding of behaviour disorders, specific factors related to extremely slow development and abnormalities of brain function might also be contributing to the development of such problems. We also pointed out that the ecological explanation was consistent with a view of behaviour problems as the result of what the person learns while interacting with the world. From this point of view, a behaviour problem is as much a learned behaviour as is an adaptive skill and can be unlearnt if the appropriate contingencies are arranged. While at present many behaviour disorders are treated pharmacologically and there is hope for significant advances in this approach in future, the best-documented techniques at present are behavioural.

Most of this chapter, then, is given over to descriptions of programmes using behaviour modification techniques aimed at eliminating behaviour problems in individuals who are profoundly retarded and multiply impaired. Since a variety of such techniques are employed, we will first note what these are and describe their main features. For those hoping to use such approaches, further familiarisation through the literature and live demonstrations are called for. Progress in the use of pharmacological intervention in conjunction with behavioural techniques has also been made in recent years, a topic that will be dealt with in Volume 3 of this series.

Behavioural Approaches to Problems

Both Schroeder, Mulick and Schroeder (1979) and Kiernan (1985) have summarised the main techniques employed in eliminating behaviour problems. Here we draw on each of their accounts.

Positive Reinforcement

Schroeder *et al.* (1979) note that in some instances undesirable behaviour can be modified by making positive reinforcement available noncontingently, i.e. making reward available without specifying any particular target behaviour. One way in which this is done is through enrichment of the environment by making toys and other rewarding experiences available. Such an approach has received little study, and it is important to note that it could never be regarded as a general cure-all since as we shall see quite different factors can maintain the same type of behaviour in two individuals. Horner (1980) describes one application of this approach and in our discussion of the functional analysis of behaviour disorders below we will note another in more detail (Iwata, Dorsey, Slifer, Bauman and Richman 1982). With respect to the prevention of behaviour problems in the first place, design of suitable environments early in development is a major priority for those working with children who are profoundly retarded and multiply impaired.

Withdrawal of Reinforcement

If we have established that a particular piece of undesirable behaviour is maintained by contingent positive reinforcement, then a learning-based approach to its elimination entails the removal of that reinforcement. Removal of reinforcement leading to the disappearance of a behaviour is referred to as 'extinction'.

There are several problems associated with the use of extinction procedures. First, it is often difficult to identify what the reinforcer is that is maintaining the behaviour, particularly if the event is only occurring intermittently. Second, withdrawal of reinforcement often leads to an initial increase in the behaviour. Where a behaviour involves injury to self or another this can result in acceleration of the behaviour and accentuated damage. Third, the number of times the behaviour can occur before extinction is complete can run to several thousand occasions, again, an unacceptable state of affairs with more serious behaviours. Both points 2 and 3 raise serious ethical issues for staff attempting to implement these procedures. Fourth, the nature of the reinforcement may be such that it is not readily amenable to intervention through withdrawal of reinforcement, most notably in the case of sensory reinforcement resulting from self-stimulatory activity.

The technique of *time-out* also involves the withdrawal of reinforcement. Schroeder *et al.* (1979) describe several different ways in which this can be achieved: first, by allowing the person to remain in the situation, e.g. the classroom, but differentially attending to desirable and undesirable behaviours; second, withdrawing oneself from the person's environment contingent on the undesirable behaviour; third, what they call exclusion time-out, i.e. not permitting the person to participate in activities in which the reinforcement leading to the problem behaviour is available; fourth, withdrawing the person and placing him or her in seclusion where it is assumed the reinforcement is no longer available; fifth, Schroeder *et al.* refer to 'contingent restraint time-out' in which the undesirable behaviour is prevented contingently, i.e. the restraint to the person is introduced following occurrence of the behaviour. This final procedure would be considered 'punishment' by many authors.

Punishment

The process of extinction described above does not involve any definite event after the person has produced the undesirable behaviour — just the withholding of the reinforcing event. In contrast, punishment entails something definite happening, such as a loud 'No!' or some other event considered to be aversive. The intention with punishment is actively to suppress the undesirable behaviour. Schroeder *et al.* list the aversive events employed most as: physical stimuli (e.g. slapping or tickling), loud noises, unpleasant smells, contingent physical restraint (physically stopping the behaviour each time it occurs), electric shocks, sometimes euphemistically referred to as 'electric stimulation' and facial screening.

In passing, we should point out that the status of time-out with respect to the distinction drawn between punishment and extinction is not clear. In time-out a specific event does follow the unacceptable behaviour though this may not in itself be regarded as aversive, e.g. the act of removing the person from a room. Some authorities, however, have suggested that, at least in some cases, time-out can be regarded as a punishment procedure.

Avoidance learning can also be employed in conjunction with punishment. Thus, pairing a signal such as 'No!' with the punishing stimulus can eventually lead to a transfer of control by which the 'No!' itself will lead the client to cease responding to avoid the punishment.

Ethical concerns with regard to use of punishment are a major consideration, though these are equally relevant to the other procedures, such as extinction, where a behaviour may be protracted and not diminish for a long period of time. Apart from following the usual procedures for gaining clearance on the ethical acceptability of the intervention, practitioners must also ensure that the programme is adequately monitored. With respect to monitoring, the reader's attention is drawn to Iwata *et al.*'s (1982) account of the procedures they developed to ensure the well-being of their clients was safeguarded while they observed, but did not intervene with, self-injurious behaviours.

There is little doubt that in many instances the use of punishment procedures is highly effective and in many cases endures for an appreciable time. The primary limitation that has emerged is the failure to generalise to situations other than the training context.

Overcorrection

This procedure was developed initially by Foxx and Azrin (1972) and consists of two main components, restitution and positive practice. Restitution entails the individual making good what disruption or damage he or she has brought about. Positive practice entails repeatedly carrying out a behaviour which is incompatible with the unacceptable behaviour. As Schroeder *et al.* point out, this is a complex technique involving feedback, time-out developing compliance, punishing noncompliance, reinforcing alternative behaviours and fading guidance.

Results on the effectiveness of this approach, and indeed, on which of the components are the effective ones, are conflicting. Nevertheless, we describe below some programmes employing overcorrection with people who are profoundly retarded and multiply impaired with some measure of success.

Differential Reinforcement Techniques

A number of approaches have been devised which aim to reinforce behaviours other than the unacceptable behaviour, thus leading to a reduction of the unacceptable behaviour.

Differential Reinforcement of Other Behaviour. One of the frequently cited techniques does not actually involve reinforcement of an alternative behaviour but reinforcement for withholding the unacceptable behaviour for a period of time. For example, reinforcement would be given at the end of a 30-second period if the behaviour had not occurred. Emission of the response during that time would reset the clock for a further 30-second period. In some respects the Differential Reinforcement of Other Behaviour (DRO) procedure is comparable to time-out and is probably most effective when used in conjunction with another technique such as time-out itself or punishment.

Differential Reinforcement of Alternative or Incompatible Behaviour. When reinforcement of a specified response other than the unacceptable behaviour is employed, the technique is referred to as Differential Reinforcement of Alternative Behaviour (DRA). If the response selected for reinforcement is incompatible with the unacceptable behaviour, the technique is referred to as Differential Reinforcement of Incompatible

Behaviour (DRI). For example, reinforcement of hands on play material is incompatible with hands on eyes. Alternatively, the response selected for reinforcement may be compatible with the unacceptable behaviour (DRC), such as hands on toys being compatible with head banging. DRI procedures are obviously the logical choice, though there is little experimental information on the relative value of reinforcing incompatible versus compatible behaviours.

Differential Reinforcement of Low Rate of Behaviour. Finally, a schedule referred to as DRL, Differential Reinforcement of Low Rate of Behaviour, may be employed. Here the unacceptable behaviour itself is reinforced, but only after it had not been emitted for some preset period of time. This interval can be progressively increased, leading eventually to a substantial reduction in the frequency of emission of the response.

Kiernan (1985) points out that whether a DRO, DRA or DRL schedule is employed will depend upon the particular circumstances of treatment and what other responses available to the client will have to be taken into account. He advocates the use of differential reinforcement techniques in conjunction with other procedures designed to reduce unacceptable behaviour.

Even a more thorough description of these techniques and their use would probably leave the reader with the basic question, 'How do I decide which technique to use and when?'. There is, in fact, no simple answer to this question, and it is only recently that much attention has been given to procedures that will enable the practitioner to make other than arbitrary decisions. The starting point for determining which techniques to use will be through an analysis of the conditions under which the unacceptable behaviour is displayed and the function the behaviour serves.

Functional Analysis

Murphy (1985) notes three approaches to undertaking such a functional analysis. The first entails careful observation of both the antecedent and consequent events and conditions under which the behaviour is displayed. The programme would emerge from this observation phase in a relatively natural way, in that the procedures used would involve systematic changes to the antecedent and consequent events. Such a procedure is time-consuming and Murphy's second suggestion involves the use of a simple questionnaire on the conditions surrounding the occurrence of the behaviour such as that produced by Durand and Crimmins (1984). Third, the environment of the individual can be systematically altered to see if there are any correlated changes in the behaviour of the person.

Iwata *et al.* (1982) report an excellent example of this last approach. They studied self-injurious behaviour in nine clients, five of whom were profoundly retarded and two of whom were clearly profoundly retarded and multiply impaired. The younger of these (Chronological Age (CA) 5 years 10 months, Mental Age (MA) 8–12 months) had congenital rubella syndrome, cerebral palsy and visual and hearing impairments. The second (CA 17 years 2 months, MA 15–24 months), also had congenital rubella syndrome with mild cerebral palsy. For these and other clients, four experimental situations were devised: (i) Social disapproval: here a situation stimulating the natural environment was devised. When the client commenced self-injurious behaviour (SIB), the experimenter showed disapproval (e.g. 'Don't do that!'). The hypothesis was that such attention might be reinforcing and increase the rate of SIB. (ii) Academic demand: here the experimenter sat with the client guiding him or her through various academic tasks (e.g. completing a wooden puzzle). Success was praised, but the occurrence of SIB led to the experimenter turning away from the client. The hypothesis here was that SIB might be produced to effect just such an escape from academic demands and would therefore be negatively reinforced by the withdrawal of attention. (iii) Unstructured play: here toys were available and the client was free to do what he or she wished. The situation was similar to Horner's (1980) enriched environment. SIB was ignored but periods in which there was no SIB were socially reinforced. The condition served as a control in which stimulating material was available, appropriate behaviour was reinforced and no demands were made. (iv) Alone: the person was alone in an unstimulating environment without toys or experimenter. The function of this environment was to see if SIB increased perhaps, as in the case of stereotyped behaviour, as a means of increasing stimulation.

One main conclusion that emerged from this functional analysis was that SIB served quite different functions for different groups of clients, i.e. any given condition might lead to an increase or decrease in SIB depending on the individual. In one pattern, the unstructured play situation lead to relatively low SIB. In a second, SIB was exhibited only in the high demand situation. A fourth pattern was one in which SIB occurred only when social disapproval was in effect. For the older of the two individuals we described above, SIB was greatest in the alone condition, i.e. he fell in pattern two. For the younger boy, however, no clear effect of any condition emerged with SIB remaining high in all conditions. Clearly further functional analysis involving manipulation of the conditions would here be called for. Given the degree of physical and sensory impairment in this child, it is possible that some intrinsic factors were maintaining SIB which were insensitive to the fairly gross environmental manipulations employed.

In reality, a period of observation followed by such experimental variations would produce the ideal functional analysis, with the explanation of what was maintaining the behaviour being further refined during the intervention phase.

Dealing with Specific Problems

If we adopted a strict criterion of considering only studies of behaviour problems which involved people who are profoundly retarded and multiply impaired, we find that the majority fall within the overall category described above on the basis of Nihira's work as 'Personal Maladaptation'. In particular the behaviours of concern are concentrated in his groups 4 and 5, i.e. 'Destructive behaviour towards property or self' and 'Stereotyped or hyperactive behaviour'. In particular, self-injurious behaviour and stereotyped behaviour figure large. In the following we will consider thse two types of behaviour as representing Nihira's Group 4 and Group 5 problems in the Personal Maladaptation area and describe the application of techniques covered above to each.

Self-injurious Behaviour

In a situation where it is not yet possible to give an *exact* definition of what in general constitutes a behaviour problem, it is inevitable that we will not be able to define precisely what a self-injurious or stereotyped behaviour consists of. With respect to SIB, Schroeder, Mulick and Rojahn (1980) point out that there is as yet no agreed definition of which behaviours should be included in the class of SIB behaviours. A definition based on obvious physical injury to the body does not cover less obvious progressive damage resulting from ingesting inappropriate substances through pica.

We should not, therefore, at present draw any hard and fast rule with regard to SIB as to which behaviours fall within this definition. Instead, inappropriate behaviours should be studied and the relations between them considered.

Among such behaviours Schroeder *et al.* (1980) include:

> Head banging
> Biting self
> Scratching self
> Gouging self
> Pinching self
> Pulling out own hair

As well as:

> Pica
> Mouthing and sucking
> Ruminative vomiting
> Coprophagy
> Aerophagia
> Polydipsia

Closely related behaviours (i.e. those frequently occurring in combination with the above) are the stereotypic responses of:

> Body rocking
> Head and torso weaving
> Hand and finger waving

With respect to the first two SIB categories, Schroeder *et al.* suggest that the first list, beginning with head banging, should be viewed as consisting of social behaviours because they are publicly obvious and likely to be maintained by social reinforcement. In contrast, those in the list starting 'pica' are more likely to be maintained by sensory consequences as part of the consummatory act. However, while behaviours in each group tend to occur together, it cannot be assumed that either class is uniquely maintained by a single type of reinforcement as we shall see. Social and/or sensory reinforcement can be involved in maintaining any given behaviour in either group.

Positive Reinforcement. As we have seen, the use of positive reinforcement in order to reduce SIB is based on the assumption that the consequence of SIB, while reinforcing in itself, is less reinforcing than some alternative stimulus available in the environment. Bailey and Meyerson (1970) clearly demonstrated this approach as a means of treatment with a boy who was profoundly retarded and nonambulant, and who chewed his hand and hit his head or leg against the bars of his crib. Two conditions were used. In one a press on a lever initiated six seconds of vibration, an event previously established as reinforcing. In the other, continuous vibration was available noncontingently, i.e the boy did not have to make a response to receive vibration.

Under the contingent vibration condition which the authors consider incompatible with SIB, an increase in lever pressing was associated directly with a decrease in SIB. This condition, of course, could also be described as Differential Reinforcment of Incompatible Behaviour, i.e. a DRI schedule. What was of special interest, however, was the observation that under the noncontingent vibration condition, SIB decreased even more, a true 'positive reinforcement available' effect. The authors comment that this demonstration is quite compatible with a view of SIB as an attempt to obtain sensory stimulation in conditions where this is highly restricted.

Bailey and Meyerson's (1970) demonstration is a relatively simple one, and there would be little difficulty in attempting to replicate it in a conventional classroom situation. The same applies to a more recent and extensive study by Favell, McGimsey and Schell (1982) with six young people who were profoundly retarded and multiply impaired. In these cases, preliminary analysis had suggested that the function of SIB was neither to gain or escape attention, but was essentially sensory in nature.

The first participant, Jim, was profoundly retarded, blind and semi-ambulant, and he chewed and sucked his hand. The intervention consisted of tying preferred toys to his wheelchair tray top. This was followed by reinforcing Jim for toy play in which he did not bring the toys to his mouth. In the first intervention condition, mouthing his hands was followed by mouthing the toys, a behaviour which under the reinforcement condition gave way to true play, i.e. vigorous movement of the toy by his ear, an appropriate activity for a visually impaired individual.

The next two participants engaged in eye poking. Both were profoundly retarded and visually impaired though with some light vision. Both poked their eyes or inserted a finger into the periorbital cavity. Again, 'toys available' was the main intervention condition with adult intervention to bring one individual into contact with the toys. For him, contact with toys successfully suppressed SIB and under this condition suppression was maintained for several months. A resurgence of eye poking that occurred subseqeuntly was attributed to a serious degeneration in available vision and a new treatment programme was devised. The other young man responded to the intervention programme with a decrease in eye poking when visual toys were made available. It is interesting to note that when nonvisual toys were available, eye poking occurred at a considerably higher level than when visual toys, e.g. a prism, were available.

The final group of young people exhibited pica, chewing and swallowing inappropriate material in a way that was potentially life threatening. All were profoundly retarded, two in wheelchairs and one able to walk only with help. Pica was reduced by presentation of toys which the participants began to chew. When appropriate toy play was reinforced such play duly increased. Presentation of popcorns, which the participants chewed for some time, also decreased pica, suggesting that oral engagement was more important than manual engagement. Following the study, suppression of pica continued, though if less chewable toys were substituted, pica again occurred.

This study emphasises how important it is to analyse the environmental conditions in relation to the nature of the person's behaviour and impairments. This point is again illustrated in Lockwood and Bourland's (1982) study of SIB in two young people who were profoundly retarded and multiply impaired. Here the importance of providing toys suitable for gripping and chewing is noted, and the greater effectiveness of having them attached (by elastic) in front of the person demonstrated an arrangement that obviously leads to less likelihood that the toys will fall to the floor or be thrown away.

All the studies indicated above point to SIB as a self-stimulatory activity for these particular young people, a behaviour that can be overcome when positively reinforcing sensory alternatives are available. Using such techniques, SIB does not disappear permanently, the appropriate environmental conditions having to be maintained. The techniques work across a wide range of distinct SIBs, ranging from those involving direct physical injury to pica. They point not only towards the design of appropriate environments when SIB has developed, but to early intervention in which at-risk children, i.e. those who are retarded, visually and/or physically impaired, are given sources of stimulation that prevent inappropriate behaviours developing.

Withdrawal of Reinforcement.

(a) Extinction. The use of extinction procedures implies, of course, that through observation or functional analysis we have identified the events that are maintaining the unacceptable behaviour. In the studies we have just reviewed, sensory reinforcement was judged as the maintaining consequence, though in other situations such consequences may well be social, resulting from the giving of attention contingent on the SIB. In the example we have chosen to show the use of an extinction procedure,

sensory consequences were again judged to be the effective events. Indeed, where SIB is maintained by social reinforcement the applicability of extinction is open to question. Bruhl, Fielding, Joyce, Peters and Wieseler (1982) comment on their own programme:

> Not only would extinction programs have been a medical risk to these residents, they would have been behaviorally unsound. Staff intervention would have occurred on a thinner schedule which, if reinforcing, would have made the behavior more resistant to deceleration than it had been prior to program implementation. (pp. 215–16)

Rincover and Devany (1982) considered three children who were profoundly retarded (though no indication is given of the presence of additional impairments). Brian was 4 years and 3 months and repeatedly banged his head on walls, floors and furniture. Sara was 4 years 6 months and seriously scratched her face with her finger nails. David was 4 years old and exhibited head banging similar to that of Brian.

In all three cases the rationale for treatment was to eliminate sensory reinforcement by interposing some shock-absorbing material between the child and the physical environment. In the case of Brian this was a padded helmet, for Sara, thin dish-washing gloves and for David, padded matting. The important point to note is that, in introducing these devices, it was not intended that they should act as permanent buffers between the child and the physical environment, but that they should eliminate sensory reinforcement. In all three cases the SIB reduced to virtually zero with introduction of the devices. Following maintenance of this reduction to a preset criterion, the special devices were faded out. In the case of the helmet and gloves this was achieved by removing them for short periods of time and increasing the duration as the child withheld SIB. The mat was faded by decreasing its thickness by removing layers from it. The training and fading parts of this study took three to four weeks and the children were still not showing SIB three to seven months later. The studies were carried out in the children's classroom and as with the earlier work on environmental enrichment, offer a readily implementable strategy to those responsible on a day to day basis.

(b) Time-out. In introducing techniques for reducing unacceptable behaviours, we included time-out with extinction as an approach involving the removal of reinforcement. Elsewhere we note that some writers see the approach as entailing punishment, i.e. the activity of implementing the time-out procedure and the effect of being timed out are considered

aversive. Here we will emphasise examples in which removal of the source of reinforcement appears to be paramount.

Schroeder, Mulick and Schroeder (1979) describe an unpublished study by Williams, Schroeder and Rojahn (1978) involving SIB and stereotyped behaviour in four boys who were profoundly retarded (though no details are given of other impairments). Four different environments were involved: (i) One in which the environment was enriched and with an adult present who reinforced behaviour contingently. (ii) One in which the environment was enriched but the adult neutral. (iii) One in which the environment was impoverished but the adult reinforced contingently. (iv) One in which the environment was impoverished and the adult neutral. A boy would be removed contingent on SIB for 30 seconds with a 10-second requirement that he refrain from SIB before release. The most effective condition was removal from the enriched environment with the reinforcing adult present; the least effective, the impoverished environment with neutral adult. The other two conditions occupied an intermediate position. Though this study does not remove the possibility that the time-out condition itself had some aversive properties, it does show that when we refer to 'time-out' we are under these circumstances referring to 'time-out from positive reinforcement'.

In their extensive programme concerned with SIB, described more fully in the following section on punishment, Bruhl *et al.* (1982) employed other forms of time-out procedure that we noted earlier in our general description of the approach. In contrast to the traditional exclusion procedure described above, SIB was dealt with by placing the individual in a standing box originally designed to enable physically handicapped people to remain upright. This was positioned in the household day area and was large enough for the person to stand comfortably without the danger of falling. The procedure was used particularly for head-banging in a tantrum-like way and the time spent in the box was from 5 to 10 minutes. This procedure is an example of what Schroeder *et al.* (1979) refer to as 'contingent restraint time-out' (p. 237). For non-tantrum SIB behaviour, reinforcement was removed by withdrawal of staff attention and other reinforcing stimuli for periods of 5 to 10 minutes. This approach is comparable to time-out methods one and three described by Schroeder *et al.* (1979) above (p. 236–7). Though these methods were employed with young people who were profoundly retarded, no description is given of their application in individual cases or of their effectiveness.

Punishment. The use of punishment techniques is now invariably seen as a last resort by those dealing with unacceptable behaviours, even where these involve life-threatening behaviour. In an extensive study of SIB, Bruhl *et al.* (1982) point out that for all 18 of their clients, the starting point for programming entailed the use of positive reinforcement, differential reinforcement of other behaviours and adjunct treatment conditions of a nonaversive nature. Given that this programming involved a 16 hour day intervention, failure to significantly affect the SIB of an individual pointed towards use of aversive methods such as time-out or punishment. Several different criteria led to this outcome depending on the particular individual. Among reasons given for moving to an aversive approach these authors note:

(i)   Intractably unco-operative behaviour and insurmountable resistance to programming.

(ii) Increased SIB in response to nonaversive programming.

(iii) Intractable self-restraint (e.g. client wrapping self in towel) preventing programming.

(iv) Erratic responses to programming and extended stay in programme.

(v)   Sudden increase in SIB following sustained improvement.

(vi) Failure to show any improvement either in general programme work or SIB.

(vii) Failure to heal damage to face as a result of SIB.

(viii) In case of self-induced vomiting, development of life-threatening situation.

(ix) Failure of mildly aversive techniques, e.g. squirting water on forehead.

Among those failing to respond to nonaversive programmes were three young people who were clearly profoundly retarded, though no specific information is given on additional impairments. The authors emphasise that despite the decision to employ aversive techniques, the nonaversive procedures were also maintained and a generally positive and benign regime was maintained throughout the aversive programme. The main aversive stimulus was electric skin shock (ESS). This was found to be most effective in its application when the electrodes were attached to the client and the shock administered by remote control. This was found to be safer and easier to administer than through use of direct contact with a prod, and was also more effective in producing generalisation throughout the residential unit.

ESS was applied when the individual exhibited the unacceptable behaviour, i.e. contingent on SIB. For RB this was head banging on the wall and hitting himself; for LG banging her head on the wheelchair and floor and hitting herself; and for KI head banging on the wall and hitting himself. The response to the treatment was 'immediate and dramatic' and was sustained for one to two years with the help of booster ESSs. The authors also report on dramatic changes in the personality of these people: 'Without exception, all these individuals who (prior to the use of ESS) were withdrawn, apprehensive, negative and irritable, uncooperative and resistant to programming, became more relaxed and were in a better mood. Frequently they were seen laughing and smiling. RB and LG became quite affectionate toward staff' (p. 247). Improvements in eye contact and responsiveness to programmes in self-help were found. Obvious improvements in physical well-being were noted and no negative side effects are reported.

Hogg (1982) reported the effectiveness of 'lemon juice therapy' in suppressing self-induced vomiting by a girl with profound retardation and physical impairments. The girl was punished for thrusting her fingers into her mouth by squirting lemon juice into her mouth through a disposable syringe. In addition to the presence of vomit in her mouth, two communicative behaviours thought to indicate distress and holding the teacher's hands were also recorded. The lemon juice was found to suppress but not eliminate both fingers in the mouth and concomitantly vomit in the mouth. The child showed an increase in hand-holding as the hands in mouth behaviour decreased and communicative behaviours varied in relation to prevailing conditions. Maintenance of the effects would have had to be specifically targeted in the procedure, by, for example, extending the procedures into the home. One of the strengths of this study was that the procedure was effectively implemented by the class teacher within the classroom.

Overcorrection. Use of an overcorrection technique to eliminate SIB with an individual who was profoundly retarded and multiply impaired is described by Johnson, Baumeister, Penland and Inwald (1982). The woman involved was 20 years old, profoundly retarded, nonambulatory and with limited vision. Among her unacceptable behaviours were hitting her face and head with her fists, banging her head on the arm of her wheelchair and a variety of stereotypies. A positive practice over-correction procedure was used, entailing repeated movements of the woman's hand to a position above her head for one minute. When a target SIB was noted, the trainer shouted 'No!' and directed the woman's hands in this way repeating the command 'Up!' When hands were maintained above her head, then physical guidance was faded. Of particular interest here was whether targeting a given behaviour, i.e. self-hit, had any effect upon a second SIB, hand-mouthing, or on the stereotypies. We will deal with this aspect of the study towards the end of the chapter where we consider the effect of intervention on concomitant behaviours.

Application of the overcorrection procedure led to reduction of self-hitting to zero and withdrawal of overcorrection resulted in its increase. Similarly, introduction and withdrawal of overcorrection for hand-mouthing led to a decline of the behaviour followed by its reinstatement. Though these authors regard overcorrection as a punishment technique, it may be seen that the nature of the positive practice, hands above head, was by no means a harsh procedure and indeed, one that the woman learnt to maintain without prompts during treatment.

Differential Reinforcement Techniques. We have described above a variety of procedures for reinforcing behaviours other than the target behaviour, noting that DRA schedules (Differential Reinforcement of Alternative Behaviours) could be effected through both reinforcement of behaviours that are incompatible with the target behaviour (DRI) or are compatible (DRC). Such procedures are to be contrasted with DRO schedules in which reinforcement is not given for a specific behaviour but for withholding the unacceptable target response for a sufficient period of time (DRO).

Azrin, Besalel and Wisotek (1982) have compared DRO and DRI schedules in relation to SIB, one of their participants being a 20 year old man who was profoundly retarded, blind and had cerebral palsy (Developmental level 0.9 years). His self-injurious behaviour entailed hitting his own nose, forehead and chin until they were swollen and cut.

The DRO procedure consisted of reinforcing the man following a preset interval in which no SIB had been performed. Thus social and edible reinforcement was given after 5 seconds as long as self-injury had not occurred. This duration was progressively increased as various time criteria were reached.

The DRI interval followed a similar pattern, but here reinforcement was given for the first appropriate behaviour (whether play or social) that occurred after a preset interval.

A further technique was introduced termed as interruption. This consisted of intervening when the man began to engage in SIB, interrupting the episode for two minutes by guiding his hands to his lap. This procedure was evaluated on its own and in conjunction with DRI, i.e. following interruption the man was reinforced for withholding SIB for a preset time interval.

Of these various approaches, DRO, DRI and DRI plus interruption, the last was by far the most effective, reducing SIB to a quarter of the level under the other two techniques. This technique was effective in both the class and living situations. The authors comment that interruption alone was also effective, though perhaps because it immediately followed the DRI plus interruption condition.

Singh, Dawson and Manning (1981b) also employed a brief period of physical restraint with a girl who was profoundly retarded, deaf and blind, and who slapped her head with her fist or palm. Again, the hands were held to the girl's side for a period of one or three minutes contingent upon SIB. While both durations were effective, one-minute holding produced a greater reduction in the behaviours. This reduction was successfully generalised across staff and settings. Singh *et al.* regarded the effectiveness of the approach as resulting from disruption of an ongoing chain of behaviour and preventing the usual reinforcing outcome.

Several studies comment on Differential Reinforcement of Compatible Behaviour (DRC) as part of wider designs. We have seen one such application in Bailey and Meyerson's (1970) study described in the section on positive reinforcement above. Johnson *et al.* (1982) also looked at the use of DRC in conjunction with overcorrection to eliminate SIB, though not with individuals who were *both* profoundly retarded *and* multiply impaired. Here decreases in the target behaviour as a result of overcorrection were paralleled by increases in the DRC behaviour. As with Bailey and Meyerson's study, this involved a press on a panel, though here a sweet was the reinforcer not vibration.

Differential Reinforcement of Other Behaviour can readily be employed with other techniques. In Lockwood and Bourland's (1982) study, described above, availability of appropriate toys led to a decrease in SIB. This trend was enhanced when a DRI contingency was introduced in which absence of SIB for a preset time interval (starting at 15 seconds and extending to 15 minutes) resulted in reinforcement of the first positive play behaviour after that period.

Stereotyped Behaviour

Similar problems are evident in attempting to provide a precise definition of stereotyped behaviour as were noted previously in relation to defining SIB. The American Psychiatric Association (1980) describes diagnostic criteria for behaviour disorders including one labelled 'stereotyped movement disorders'. This category includes recurrent involuntary, repetitive, rapid, purposeless motor movement (tics) and/or nonspasmodic, stereotyped, voluntary, purposeless movements (e.g.

head banging, rocking, hand waving). A list of sub-types is given including transient tic disorder, chronic motor tic disorder, Tourette's disorder, atypical tic disorder and atypical stereotyped movement disorder. A simpler definition given in LaGrow and Repp (1984 p. 595) describes stereotypic responding as 'repetitious acts, with invariant typography and no apparent function'.

The essential features are the repetition and lack of apparent function, although as many reviews of the origins and causes of stereotyping have pointed out (e.g. Baumeister 1978), certain stereotyped behaviours may be functional to the individual concerned. For example, as noted in Volume 1, Chapters 4 and 8, stereotypical behaviour in the visual modality, such as eye poking, may provide visual stimulation for people with impaired vision. The inclusion in the first definition given above of references to 'involuntary' and 'rapid' movements may apply to some, rather than all, stereotyped behaviour for as we shall see, studies have demonstrated that behaviours can sometimes be selectively reduced under certain conditions. Furthermore, the notion that such behaviour is involuntary may reflect the psychoanalytic approach taken by the American Psychiatric Association.

In Volume 1, Chapter 4 we noted that many stereotyped behaviours occur in normally developing infants and that it is the frequency of these behaviours and their persistence into later childhood and adulthood that lead to them being defined as a problem. In addition, it is the unacceptable forms of stereotyped behaviour such as body rocking and head weaving that are usually defined as problems whereas more acceptable ones such as pencil tapping or foot tapping tend to pass unnoticed. Interestingly, observations might sometimes suggest that the staff working with people with mental handicap in residential settings show as many stereotyped behaviours as the residents', albeit different behaviours!

Comprehensive reviews of intervention research on stereotypic responding are provided by LaGrow and Repp (1984) and Gorman-Smith and Matson (1985). The LaGrow and Repp review specifies the studies which are concerned with people with profound retardation although details are not always included on their additional impairments. Throughout the selected review of intervention studies given below the target populations are both profoundly retarded and multiply impaired unless stated as otherwise.

Positive Reinforcement. The high frequency of stereotyped behaviours among institutionalised persons with retardation has been assumed to relate to the lack of stimulation in terms of both individual staff time and appropriate equipment in these environments. As previously noted, a major concern for parents and staff working with people with profound retardation and multiple impairment is the provision of a suitable environment. It may have been the assumption that more stimulation was required, which led to the common practice of having music and/or television constantly turned on in hospital wards. Alternatively, this may have evolved for the pleasure of the staff and to compensate for the lack of verbal feedback from noncommunicating clients. Adams, Tallon and Stangl (1980) point out that there are no data supporting the use of noncontingent music or television as a method of reducing stereotyped behaviours. In their study of four residents with profound retardation, only one of whom was multiply impaired, they compared levels of stereotypic behaviour under conditions of quiet, music on, or television on and no toys, toys, toys plus staff interaction. It was found that the levels of stereotypic behaviour were highest when the television was on and lowest when the music from a radio was playing. The authors concluded that far from livening up a drab living environment, the television may be detrimental to lower functioning residents. It was noted that discrepancies between this finding and previous studies (e.g. Forehand and Baumeister 1970) may suggest that the precise sound conditions and amount of oscillation may affect stereotypic behaviour. A former example of this point was provided by Stevens (1971) who demonstrated that the tempo of music may differentially affect the rocking behaviour of people with severe and profound retardation (who did not have multiple impairments) according to the tempo of their rocking. It was found for example that music presented at a tempo antagonistic to 'fast rockers' resulted in decreased rocking whereas the same slow tempo music increased the rocking of 'slow rockers'.

No significant differences in stereotypic behaviour were noted in this study under the various toy conditions, which again conflicts with some other studies (e.g. Horner 1980). It was noted that the residents either ignored the toys completely or used them as part of their stereotypic repertoire. The lack of changes noted under the condition in which a staff member gave instructions was considered by the authors as possibly resulting from the specific procedure used in this study, which it was thought might have accidentally reinforced the residents' stereotypic behaviour. It is inconsistent with findings from studies of the rates of disruptive and stereotypic behaviour under room management schemes (e.g. Porterfield, Blunden and Blewitt 1980) in which rates are reported to decrease during times when staff are regularly interacting with the client on tasks. However, from our description of room management schemes given in Chapter 2 of this volume, it will be apparent that the reduction of stereotyping may be as a result of the regular staff contact or may be due to the consistent positive reinforcement of other behaviours which is occurring when a scheme is in operation.

An example of a more specific adaptation of the environment, in an attempt to reduce object destruction (which sometimes occurs collaterally to stereotypical behaviours), is the use of devices to protect leisure materials reported by Marks and Wade (1981). Objects such as musical instruments, books and drawing materials were made available continuously, without specific supervision, by sliding them into metal frames bolted to the tables. Clients who were severely and profoundly retarded (no information given on additional impairments) were reinforced for any contact with the materials that was not destructive. The outcome of the study is reported in terms of a reduction in the number of objects destroyed rather than in terms of frequencies of client behaviours. It is suggested that this type of device can counteract the need to place individuals in barren settings for the protection of self or others.

Some other environmental variables that have been considered in relation to rates of stereotypical behaviour include the density of people and amount of space available. Warren and Burns (1970) found that stereotypical behaviours occurred more frequently when the children who were severely and profoundly retarded but not multiply impaired, were placed in their cribs during rest periods, than at times when they were out of their cribs. The authors postulated various possible explanations such as boredom and lack of access to staff which occurred when the children were in the cribs.

Withdrawal of Reinforcement.

(a) Extinction. We described the way in which extinction procedures have been used to reduce and eliminate SIBs by removing the reinforcing properties of the behaviours through the use of devices such as padding. Another type of extinction procedure can be labelled 'escape extinction' which involves eliminating opportunities for the individual to escape from an aversive stimulus. A common difficulty met with while teaching new skills concerns clients who continually escape from the instruction by leaving their chairs, running off, etc. Carr, Newsom and Binkoff (1980) describe a 14 year old child called Bob with a social age of 3.3 years (no reference is made to additional impairments) whose teachers complained that he had become totally unmanageable (scratching, kicking, biting or hitting) when even a minimal demand, such

as having to sit in a chair, was made. They initiated an 'escape extinction' procedure with Bob to eliminate his aggression during teaching sessions and to initiate an imitation training programme. During the sessions Bob was secured to the chair with a seat belt thus eliminating any opportunity to escape. Sessions were extended if necessary to avoid ending them during incidences of aggressive behaviour. In session 22 the seatbelt was removed and in session 25 the experimenter began to remove the protective clothing (heavy duty coat and rubber gloves) he had been wearing. In session 32 imitation training began.

Initially the number of aggressive responses remained high but by session 4 it had markedly dropped and by session 6 was limited to one or two acts per session. On certain sessions negative reinforcement was introduced allowing Bob to leave the chair for one minute following aggressive acts. During these sessions the aggressive responses rose again, in the first negative reinforcement session to 1,625 responses! Each time extinction was reintroduced aggression dropped to a near-zero level. By the end of the experiment (session 39) Bob was correctly responding on a two-way motor imitative discrimination 97 per cent of the time. The use of escape extinction therefore not only eliminated Bob's aggressive behaviour but made him able to tolerate high frequencies of demands.

(b) *Time-out.* We described above a number of different ways in which time-out can be used. The first approach mentioned was that in which the person remains in the same place but reinforcement is given differentially to desirable and undesirable behaviour. Davis, Wieseler and Hanzel (1980) describe an adult with profound retardation (no details given of additional impairments) who had a long history of ruminatory behaviour and out-of-seat behaviour, defined as sitting or lying on the floor, twirling, hopping and pacing around the room. Sessions took place half an hour after each meal and consisted of seating the client in the room with a cassette recorder playing instrumental bluegrass music. The music was turned off for a short time after rumination or until the client reseated himself after each occurrence of out-of-seat behaviour. Other phases of the study involved introducing a verbal cue 'No' when rumination began, either coupled with the time-out condition or on its own.

It was found that although the verbal cue and the time-out conditions each reduced ruminations considerably, a near-zero rate of rumination was only achieved by combining both procedures. Out-of-seat behaviours dropped as a result of the time-out contingency from occurring for half of the 12 minute session time to less than one minute of it.

In practice, many studies dealing with stereotypic or aggressive behaviours combine procedures involving the withdrawal of reinforcement with reinforcement of other, alternative or incompatible behaviours. There would appear to be ethical concern about extinguishing the few behaviours some clients with profound retardation and multiple impairments display, without replacing them with any other behaviours.

Punishment. Punishment encompasses many varied procedures including verbal or physical stimuli, use of unpleasant smells or tastes, facial screening, contingent physical restraint and electric shocks. Punishment procedures appear to have become somewhat less commonly used probably due to the difficulties in justifying them ethically for the treatment of stereotypies which unlike SIBs are rarely life threatening.

Facial screening has become a more commonly used technique since the mid-1970s to reduce undesirable behaviours. The procedure is more socially and ethically acceptable than electric shocks, and the apparatus more portable, easier to use and can be administered by anyone with minimal training. The technique's major disadvantage is that it requires one-to-one therapy sessions, though this applies to most of the procedures which we are considering here.

Singh, Winton and Dawson (1982) describe the use of facial screening with an adult who was profoundly retarded (no information on additional impairments is given) who had a two year history of screaming with no known organic cause. Sessions took place at three different locations within the resident's ward and at the start of each session a large terry-cloth bib was tied around the resident's neck. Whenever the resident screamed, the bib was placed quickly over her face and held firmly at the back of the head for one minute without restricting breathing. Screaming was eliminated in all three settings within a few days. Very few screaming responses occurred in the sixth month maintenance phase, during which time all ward staff implemented contingent facial screening. During the sixth month follow-up after the maintenance phase had ended, screaming occurred less than twice per month.

Contingent physical restraint is another procedure that is relatively straightforward to administer and has been noted to be effective in some studies. For example, Reid, Tombaugh and Heuvel (1981) introduced physical restraint to seven residents who were profoundly retarded (no information is given on additional impairments) who body rocked at the rate of at least 100 rocks (each defined as one forward and backward movement of the upper body) per 20-minute period. Two treatment procedures were used: the restraint up and the restraint down. Each resident was restrained either in the upright position (restraint up) or in the bent-over position (restraint down) for one minute during the occurrence of each body rock in the 20-minute session. Three residents received the restraint up procedure and four the restraint down procedure for 10 sessions, after which the type of restraint was reversed between residents for a further ten sessions (with a baseline phase between the two treatment phases).

The amount of body rocking was reduced for every resident and the restraint down procedure was more effective in suppressing rocking for most of the residents. Two possible explanations are given for this observed difference between the effectiveness of the procedures. The 'response topography' explanation suggests that the 'down' position is more unnatural for the resident and can therefore be more easily discriminated than the more usual 'upright' position. The alternative explanation is the 'response chaining' hypothesis which suggests that the 'down' position is in the middle of the chain of sequential responses involved in body rocking. Interrupting the response in the middle rather than at the end is considered to be more effective. One would need to compare applications of the same restraint at different times of the response sequence to confirm which explanation is valid.

Unfortunately, once restraint had been discontinued the lower levels of rocking noted during the treatment phase were not maintained for all residents. Moreover, changes in rocking behaviour had not generalised to the wards, the treatment having taken place in an experimental room. This is a common problem in punishment procedures as we suggested earlier in this chapter. Although contingent restraint is initially effective, like other forms of punishment, it does not increase adaptive behaviour but provides temporary suppression of undesirable behaviour. LaGrow and Repp (1984) argue, in line with many other writers in this field, that these procedures should therefore only be adopted when more positive methods have failed.

Overcorrection. Overcorrection has been described as 'an educative punishment procedure' (Foxx 1976 p. 54) because the individuals are taught to accept responsibility for their behaviour through the restitution procedures that require restoration of the disturbed situation in an exaggerated way. Furthermore, appropriate responses are then practised. It is perhaps the idea that this procedure teaches people to be responsible for their own behaviour that has led to its tremendous popularity. Gorman-Smith and Matson (1985) carried out a meta-analysis (statistical comparison of treatment effects across studies) of research reported on stereotypy and self-injury and found that overcorrection procedures had been used far more than any other approaches, although they were *not* the most effective.

An attempt to eliminate object transferral, defined as attempts to pass an object from hand to hand with no constructive intent, by an adult with profound retardation but who had no additional impairments, is reported by Martin, Weller and Matson (1977). The overcorrection procedure developed by Azrin, Kaplan and Foxx (1973) to reduce stereotypies with residents who were severly and profoundly retarded was used. When Mary transferred objects she was told 'No Mary' and she was instructed to hold her arms in one of three positions randomly selected, for 15 seconds. This procedure successfully reduced the stereotypical behaviour from a level of 99 per cent of the time to a level of 0.04 per cent of the time. Generalisation to other settings was reported but no long-term follow-up data were given. In this study the overcorrection procedure employed seems to have focused on the restitution with little attention given to positive practice. Was the stationary position of Mary's arms necessarily more adaptive than the object transferring behaviour being eliminated?

A clearer distinction between the restitution and positive practice procedures involved in overcorrection is apparent in Foxx's (1976) description of the reduction of stripping (which was stereotypical in that it was repetitive and nonfunctional although not in the same category of behaviour in Nihira's (1978) list (pp. 232–3). Amy was an adult with profound retardation and had physical and auditory impairments and epilepsy. She had been stripping for 40 years. The restitution part of the procedure required her to pick up her discarded clothing and to dress herself in the discarded clothes plus additional items of clothing with physical prompts where necessary. Once dressed she would be taken through the positive practice procedure involving her in assisting other residents in improving their personal appearance, including buttoning or zipping up any undone clothing, straightening crumpled or twisted clothing, assisting with the replacement of footwear and haircombing. After 40 days of treatment Amy's stripping was eliminated. She had previously been stripping an average of five times per day and had therefore been excluded from many activities such as outings, to which she was now reintroduced without any further incidents of stripping. The restitution and positive practice procedures in this example offered opportunities for the development of adaptive dressing skills and inter-action with other residents.

Problems of generalisation and maintenance have received a great deal of attention in relation to overcorrection procedures although neither of the studies reported above include much information on these aspects. Foxx and Livesay (1984) retrospectively examined overcorrection programmes over a ten-year period and concluded that the lower functioning individuals show poorer maintenance of response suppression than higher functioning ones and that certain behaviours, such as coprophagy and pica, are more difficult to suppress in the long term. In addition, many problems were noted in relation to maintaining staff behaviour. Overcorrection programmes were less likely to be reinstated than other procedures because of their complexity, staff intensity, the time and effort required by them and the requirements of monitoring involved. They suggest trying to ensure programmes are kept as short and simple as possible, with built in generalisation procedures (a point reiterated by LaGrow and Repp 1984) and should begin with the least problematic clients to enable staff to be encouraged to continue with them.

Differential Reinforcement Techniques.

(a) DRO. Differential Reinforcement of Other Behaviour (DRO) involves reinforcement for specified periods, during which the stereotypical behaviour has not occurred. This technique therefore involves reinforcing any other behaviour which occurs during the specified time whether seen as specifically adaptive or not. It has been extensively used for the reduction of stereotypical behaviours particularly in conjunction with other techniques.

An example of an application of a DRO procedure in conjunction with momentary physical restraint is provided by Barton, Repp and Brulle (1985) who report successful reduction of hand clapping, mouthing and light gazing in four students some of whom were profoundly retarded (the authors do not specify how many) and all of whom had additional impairments of vision, hearing and motor skills. The procedure involved reinforcing the student at the end of each period in which no stereotypical behaviours occurred. The length of the period was determined on the basis of each student's baseline rate of stereotypy. For example, if the student showed stereotypical behaviours initially at an average rate of once each two minutes, the DRO interval used was two minutes. The interval was then modified each day in accordance with the rate of stereotyping during the previous day.

Momentary restraint consisted of holding the students' arms by their sides in the case of hand flapping and mouthing and holding the student's head in midline in the case of light gazing. Initially, the restraint was carried out for 3 seconds but was increased to a maximum of 10 seconds if not effective over three days.

Both the DRO and momentary restraint procedures were effectively applied within the school setting and throughout the day by the teachers and aides, with a significant reduction of each student's stereotypical behaviour although none of the behaviours was eliminated. The notable feature of this study seems to have been the applicability of the procedures within the normal setting by the staff although no long-term maintenance data are given.

(b) DRA/DRI. Differential Reinforcement of Alternative or Incompatible Behaviour (DRA/DRI) is also a technique often applied in conjunction with other techniques to reduce stereotypical behaviours. McDaniel, Kocim and Barton (1984) describe a combined DRI and punishment procedure to eliminate stereotypical mouthing behaviour in Diane, a young child who was deaf-blind, hypertonic and whose cognitive abilities were described as 'very elementary'. Whenever Diane had her fingers in her mouth they were removed by a staff member who said 'No' and shook Diane's head firmly from side to side. In addition, Diane received edible reinforcements every time she touched a toy. After 11 days of treatment within the classroom her mouthing, which had taken place 97 per cent of the school day, was eliminated. No follow-up data are reported.

An example combining DRI and overcorrection is provided by Denny (1980) which involved wheelchair mobility training as an overcorrection procedure for three children with profound retardation and physical impairments who all hand-mouthed and showed a variety of other stereotypies involving their hands. The study compared applying a DRI procedure alone which consisted of social praise for two-handed toy play, with the same procedure in addition to an overcorrection procedure. This involved telling the children 'No' and prompting their hands to propel a wheelchair for one minute, each time the stereotypical behaviour occurred.

The DRI procedure alone only slightly reduced stereotypical behaviour, whereas the combined treatment resulted in a reduction to near-zero levels for all three children. These reductions were maintained on one and two month (no treatment) follow-ups. The author considered that the contingent movement of the specific body part involved in the stereotypical behaviour was responsible for the changes noted. He did not consider that the adaptive nature of the substitute behaviour (the wheelchair mobility training) contributed to the outcome, since none of the individuals actually mastered this skill during the study.

Elsewhere, Berkson (1983) has suggested that to be maximally effective, alternative behaviour procedures should provide the same class of sensory functions as that provided by the stereotypical behaviours. This may have applied in the Denny study if the individuals' stereotypical behaviour with their hands was providing them with manual tactile stimulation which might also have been provided by the wheelchair mobility training. However, if the hand-mouthing is assumed to be providing oral stimulation, this function was not served by the propelling of the wheels. Williams (1978) found that vibration as a reinforcer for the incompatible behaviour of lever pressing was more effective in reducing visually orientated stereotypies than light stimulation. In this case, sensory stimulation matched to self-stimulation was *not* preferred to that providing a different form of stimulation. Hence, it would seem important to consider both the specific parts of the body involved in the stereotypy and the form of stimulation it might be providing.

(c) DRL. The Differential Reinforcement of Low Rate Behaviour (DRL) is a much less well documented approach and the few studies reported relate to reducing disruptive behaviour in classrooms. The procedure can be applied in several ways: by reinforcing each response that occurs at more than a fixed minimum time after the previous response; by reinforcing responses that occur on average more than a fixed minimum time after the previous one; by reinforcing the individual provided there is less than a fixed maximum number of stereotypical responses throughout a session.

Singh, Dawson and Manning (1981a) provide an example of an application of the first of these three procedures, that is, reinforcing each response provided it occurs sufficiently long after the previous one. Three young adults who were profoundly retarded but *not* multiply impaired and who showed a variety of stereotypical behaviours were praised following a stereotypical response, provided the minimum fixed time of 12 seconds had passed since the previous response. If a response was given before the 12 seconds elapsed that interval was terminated and the next one begun. The next three phases of the study involved increasing the minimum time required between responses to 30 seconds, 60 seconds and 180 seconds.

Stereotypical behaviours were substantially reduced for all three people although not by any means eliminated. No follow-up data are given. The authors point out that complete suppression of these behaviours in members of institutionalised populations who have access only to minimal positive environmental stimulation does not seem ethically justifiable. LaGrow and Repp (1984), developing the same point, suggest teaching individuals to discriminate between free periods, learning periods and social periods. During free periods, self-stimulation would be accepted as an adaptive response, providing the individuals with stimulation which would not otherwise be available.

We have described above a number of different techniques applied to reduce or eliminate stereotypical behaviours in people with profound retardation and, in many cases, multiple impairments. The relative effectiveness of the various techniques across studies is reviewed fully in Gorman-Smith and Matson (1985) and LaGrow and Repp (1984). However, a few points are worth summarising here to assist practitioners in their choice of intervention techniques.

Comparing three of the major categories that we have used above, positive reinforcement procedures, punishment and differential reinforcement techniques, La Grow and Repp found that punishment was the most effective followed closely by differential reinforcement techniques and lagging well behind, positive reinforcement procedures. However, more effective than any of these three categories in isolation, were combined procedures, especially restraint with overcorrection, restraint with DRO and overcorrection with DRI. These last two have the advantage of combining positive with aversive procedures. Gorman-Smith and Matson (1985) provide some contradictory evidence to LaGrow and Repp, finding for example that DRO was more effective than DRI, whereas these latter authors noted the reverse. It is important to note, however, that Gorman-Smith and Matson's review includes studies of both stereotypical behaviours and SIBs whereas LaGrow and Repp's is limited to the former. What of particular interest emerged from the meta-analysis was that the more commonly used techniques, those of overcorrection, physical restraint and facial screening, were also the least effective!

What advice can we then offer to those embarking on programmes attempting to reduce stereotypical behaviours? First, there is little doubt that individual characteristics both of the client and of the situation are very important. A positive point to emerge from the Gorman-Smith and Matson analysis was that individuals who are profoundly retarded responded better to intervention than those with less retardation. In addition, older clients responded more positively which seems contrary to the commonly held view that younger clients who have been stereotyping for fewer years are more receptive to intervention. It will be no surprise that better gains are made with stereotypical behaviours than with SIBs and that within the stereotypies least gains are made with body rocking, which is by far the commonest behaviour.

Other Approaches

Undoubtedly the most extensively documented techniques for dealing with unacceptable behaviours are the behavioural approaches we have described above. Other evaluated strategies have been evolved, however, and we consider two main classes here. The first class involves different kinds of use of the restraining devices which have for so long been used to prevent individuals engaging in the more dangerous kinds of unacceptable behaviour. These methods are in no way inconsistent with behavioural approaches, and indeed, many elements of them explicitly use such techniques. The second class entails more general programmes of physical stimulation.

The Use of Restraint

The main physical method for dealing with the more damaging kinds of unacceptable behaviour in the past has been restraint. This can range from tying the individual's hands down so that they cannot be used for self-injury through to the use of strait-jackets. While any programme would be aimed at removing the necessity of such restraints, which can both limit the opportunity to interact with the world and can cause damage to tendons, several programmes have recently attempted to use the restraining device itself as part of the intervention. Favell, McGimsey and Jones (1978) built on the observation that for some individuals the restraining device actually comes to have positively reinforcing properties for the person. Thus, they employed restraining devices as reinforcers for increasing periods of not engaging in SIB in both children and an adult who were profoundly retarded.

Hamad, Isley and Lowry (1983) report on studies in which the restraining device has been progressively faded by, for example, gradually reducing its size, eventually leading to its elimination. In their own study they describe elimination of a restraining device and the performance of SIBs in its absence with a man who was profoundly retarded and blinded by SIB. The SIB in question involved the man hitting himself in the eyes with his knee. A brace to prevent this restrained such movement. The treatment approach involved the arrangement of conditions in which the brace was removed for 15-minute periods during the day, the number of such periods being progressively increased over the course of the programme. During these periods without the brace, massive positive reinforcement was available in contrast to the time when the brace was on. Then, the man was effectively ignored except for minimal attention during self-help activities. During the restraint-free periods, any attempt to bring his knee to his eyes was dealt with in three ways: first, behaviour incompatible with this SIB was physically guided, i.e. he was made to stand; second, the action was prevented by holding down his ankle; third, access to the reinforcers was prevented for 30 seconds. Through progressive increases in the brace-free periods the occurrence of the SIB was eliminated first in the day and then during the night.

Hamad *et al.* (1983), drawing on the studies of restraint as a reinforcer, fading of restraint and their own approach suggest the following features of a treatment strategy:

> (i) a schedule of application and removal of mechanical restraint which is contingent upon behavior; (ii) a schedule of application and removal which is programmed gradually over time; (iii) using mechanical restraint as a reinforcing consequence contingent upon appropriate behavior or the absence of SIB; (iv) requiring a brief period without SIB prior to restraint application; and (v) using additional procedures such as reinforcement of alternative/incompatible behavior or time out from positive reinforcement. (p. 216).

They add that the specific combination of treatment procedures will vary depending on the frequency of the SIB, the functional nature of the behaviour and the form the behaviour takes.

Less studied, but of some potential significance, is the activity of *self-restraint*. In Bruhl *et al.*'s (1982) project that we described above, over half the clients attempted to prevent their own SIB by restraining themselves. For example, RB, to whom we referred, pushed both arms through one arm hole of his T-shirt to prevent movement. In one of the few functional analyses of self-restraint, Silverman, Watanabe, Marshall and Baer (1984) argue that self-restraint behaviour is reinforced by escape from or avoidance of self-injury, in other words, self-restraint is negatively reinforcing. They recorded what happened to self-restraining behaviour when a child wore protective clothing, e.g. a padded helmet to prevent injury to head through hitting himself. They noted that under such a condition both hits to the head and self-restraint of his arm decreased. They argue that with the hands, or body, freed from self-restraint while protective clothing is worn, new adaptive skills can be taught, and the protective clothing gradually faded.

Sensorimotor Activities

These passive stimulation techniques involve tactile, proprioceptive and vestibular stimulation that can be achieved through self-produced activity in more able people. This was effected for three individuals who were profoundly retarded and multiply impaired through the teaching of gross motor activities by Lancioni, Smeets, Ceccarani, Capodaglio and Campanari (1984). In different measure, the three individuals engaged in SIB such as self-hitting and biting. These activities occurred as a component of tantrums that were not apparently triggered by any observable environmental event. The intervention consisted of a variety of gross motor activities that the individuals undertook during periods when they were quiet. Examples of these gross motor activities included: winding wire cords, hoses and ropes and storing them; inflating rubber tubes, cushions and other inflatable objects by means of a pump; watering trees and plants by means of a bucket; and so on. The task demands were communicated by teachers verbally or through gesture and appropriate responding positively reinforced. Sessions lasted from 15 to 20 minutes and were spread across the day, building from one or two hours at the start to three hours.

Results clearly indicate that the gross motor activities led to a marked decrease in tantrum behaviour and a decrease in the duration of any given tantrum. This did not appear to be the result of fatigue as work on other classroom tasks was not affected by tiredness. The authors favour an explanation in terms of enhanced sensory input which either substituted for the sensory consequences of tantruming, or provided sensory input that mitigated the need for such tantrums.

This study is consistent with Prescott's (1976) somatosensory theory presented in detail in Chapter 4 of Volume 1. His argument was couched in terms of the consequences of blindness leading to reduced mobility and hence lack of proprioceptive and vestibular stimulation. Reduced mobility from physical impairment and lack of stimulation to engage in movement can also lead to Prescott's reduced somatosensory experience with the result that aberrant behaviours develop. Passive or active stimulation of this system would be expected to have a beneficial effect in reducing SIB and stereotypies, and if incorporated in the curriculum at a sufficiently early stage might be expected to prevent their eventual occurrence.

Collateral Behaviours

We mentioned in our earlier discussion of definitions that certain behaviours tend to occur together. Schroeder, Mulick and Rojahn (1980), for example, point out the most frequent combination of SIBs is head banging, self-biting and self-scratching and that these can be associated with stereotypies. They note the danger of targeting just one behaviour for intervention since the rate of a second might increase and the overall effect of the intervention might be simply to rearrange the pattern of unacceptable behaviour. This is clearly illustrated in the study by Johnson *et al.* (1982) described earlier. Here overcorrection was applied to behaviours selected from self-hitting, hand-mouthing, head to chair, inappropriate vocalisation, foot banging and stereotopy in a woman who was profoundly retarded. In the first phase, self-hitting was the target behaviour. This behaviour decreased to near zero and with it hand-mouthing and inappropriate vocalisations diminished. In contrast, stereotyped behaviour increased dramatically. When overcorrection of self-hitting was terminated, this, together with hand-mouthing and inappropriate vocalisation, increased. Stereotypy dropped, though remained above the original baseline.

This study illustrates that changes in what are referred to as collateral behaviours may be positive or negative. They may all be outside the initial range of behaviour problems that are of concern. In Hogg's (1982) study on self-induced vomiting, positive social behaviours emerged with some consistency as the activity associated with target behaviour diminished. In this case the child gradually began to reach out to the teacher and hold his hands instead of putting them in her mouth. It is clearly important to ensure that a range of potentially significant behaviours are monitored during interventions aimed at reducing undesirable behaviours, and that where novel behaviours begin to emerge, attention should be paid to their development and to the course they follow.

Concluding Comment

Many of the studies described in this chapter failed to report on either generalisation of outcomes to other settings or maintenance over the longer term. Lambert, Bruwier and Cobben (1975) showed that although punishment procedures may be very effective, the consequences are situation specific and they are the most difficult procedures for the teacher to apply in the classroom. Wieseler, Hanson, Chamberlain and

Thompson (1985) have argued that lack of generalisation to other settings is due to the differences in the controlling variables across situations. The functional properties of the behavior may be different in each situation requiring a different approach in each.

Since we are operating in a climate in which the philosophy of the 'least restrictive environment' prevails for people who are profoundly retarded and multiply impaired, the selection of an intervention technique might best operate through a hierarchy of procedures, as suggested by Gorman-Smith and Matson, from positive to negative.

References

Adams, G.L., Tallon, R.J. and Stangl, J.M. (1980) 'Environmental Influences on Self-Stimulatory Behavior', *American Journal of Mental Deficiency, 85,* 171–5

American Psychiatric Association (1980) *Diagnostic and Statistical Manual of Mental Disorders, 3rd edn, DSM-111,* American Psychiatric Association, Washington, D.C.

Azrin, N.H., Besalel, V.A. and Wisotek, I.E. (1982) 'Treatment of Self-injury by a Reinforcement plus Interruption Procedure', *Analysis and Intervention in Developmental Disabilities, 2,* 105–13

Azrin, N.H., Kaplan, S.J. and Foxx, R.M. (1973) 'Autism Reversal: Eliminating Stereotyped Self-Stimulation of Retarded Individuals', *American Journal of Mental Deficiency, 78,* 241–8

Bailey, J. and Meyerson, L. (1970) 'Effect of Vibratory Stimulation on a Retardate's Self-Injurious Behaviour', *Psychological Aspects of Disability, 17,* 340

Barton, L.E., Repp, A.C. and Brulle, A.R. (1985) 'Reduction of Stereotypic Behaviours using Differential Reinforcement Procedures and Momentary Restraint', *Journal of Mental Deficiency Research, 29,* 71–9

Baumeister, A.A. (1978) 'Origins and Control of Stereotyped Movements' in C.E. Meyers (ed.), *Quality of Life in Severely and Profoundly Retarded People: Research Foundations for Improvement,* American Association on Mental Deficiency, Washington, D.C.

Berkson, G. (1983) 'Repetitive Stereotyped Behaviors', *American Journal of Mental Deficiency, 88,* 239–46

Bruhl, H.H., Fielding, L., Joyce, M., Peters, W. and Wieseler, N. (1982) 'Thirty Month Demonstration Project for Treatment of Self-injurious Behavior in Severely Retarded Individuals' in J.H. Hollis and C.E. Meyers (eds.), *Life-threatening Behavior: Analysis and Intervention,* American Association on Mental Deficiency, Washington, D.C.

Carr, E.G., Newsom, C.P. and Binkoff, J.A. (1980) 'Escape as a Factor in the Aggressive Behavior of Two Retarded Children', *Journal of Applied Behavior Analysis, 13,* 101–17

Davis, W.B., Wieseler, N.A., and Hanzel, T.E. (1980) 'Contingent Music in Management of Rumination and Out-of-Seat Behavior in a Profoundly Mentally Retarded Institutionalised Male', *Mental Retardation, 18,* 43–5

Denny, M. (1980) 'Reducing Self-Stimulatory Behavior of Mentally Retarded Persons by Alternative Positive Practice', *American Journal of Mental Deficiency, 84,* 610–15

Durand, V.M. and Crimmins, D.B. (1984) 'The Motivation Assessment Scale', cited as personal communication by G. Murphy (1985) 'Self-Injurious Behaviour in the Mentally Handicapped: An Update', *Association for Child Psychology and Psychiatry Newsletter, 7,* 2–11

Eyman, R.K. and Call, T. (1977) 'Maladaptive Behavior and Community Placement of Mentally Retarded Persons', *American Journal of Mental Deficiency, 82,* 137–44

Favell, J.E., McGimsey, J.F. and Jones, M.L. (1978) 'The Use of Physical Restraint in the Treatment of Self-Injury and as Positive Reinforcement', *Journal of Applied Behavior Analysis, 11,* 225–41

Favell, J.E., McGimsey, J.F. and Schell, R.M. (1982) 'Treatment of Self-Injury by Providing Alternate Sensory Activities', *Analysis and Intervention in Developmental Disabilities, 2,* 83–104

Forehand, R. and Baumeister, A.A. (1970) 'The Effect of Auditory and Visual Stimulation on Stereotyped Rocking Behavior and General Activity of Severe Retardates', *Journal of Clinical Psychology, 26,* 426–9

Foxx, R.M. (1976) 'The Use of Overcorrection to Eliminate the Public Disrobing (Stripping) of Retarded Women', *Behavior Research and Therapy, 14,* 53–61

Foxx, R.M. and Azrin, N.H. (1972) 'Restitution: A Method of Eliminating Aggressive-Disruptive Behavior of Retarded and Brain Damaged Patients', *Behavior Research and Therapy, 10,* 15–27

Foxx, R.M. and Livesay, J. (1984) 'Maintenance of Response Suppression Following Overcorrection: A 10–Year Retrospective Examination of Eight Cases', *Analysis and Intervention in Developmental Disabilities, 4,* 65–79

Gorman-Smith, D. and Matson, J.L. (1985) 'A Review of Treatment Research for Self-Injurious and Stereotyped Responding', *Journal of Mental Deficiency Research, 29,* 295–308

Hamad, C.D., Isley, E. and Lowry, M. (1983) 'The Use of Mechanical Restraint and Response Incompatability to Modify Self-Injurious Behavior: A Case Study', *Mental Retardation, 21,* 213–17

Hogg, J. (1982) 'Reduction of Self-Induced Vomiting in a Multiply Handicapped Girl by "Lemon Juice Therapy" and Concomitant Changes in Social Behaviour', *British Journal of Clinical Psychology, 21,* 227–8

Horner, R.D. (1980) 'The Effects of an Environmental "Enrichment" Program on the Behavior of Institutionalised Profoundly Retarded Children', *Journal of Applied Behavior Analysis, 13,* 473–92

Iwata, B.A., Dorsey, M.F., Slifer, K.J., Bauman, K.E. and Richman, G.S. (1982) 'Towards a Functional Analysis of Self-Injury', *Analysis and Intervention in Developmental Disabilities, 2,* 3–20

Johnson, W.L., Baumeister, A.A., Penland, M.J. and Inwald, C. (1982) 'Experimental Analysis of Self-Injurious, Stereotypic, and Collateral Behavior of Retarded Persons: Effects of Overcorrection and Reinforcement of Alternative Responding', *Analysis and Intervention in Developmental Disabilities, 2,* 41–66

Kiernan, C.C. (1985) 'Behaviour Modification' in A.M. Clarke, A.D.B. Clarke and J.M. Berg (eds.), *Mental Deficiency: The Changing Outlook,* 4th edn. Methuen, London

LaGrow, S.J. and Repp, A.C. (1984) 'Stereotypic Responding: A View of Intervention Research', *American Journal of Mental Deficiency, 88,* 595–609

Lambert, J.L., Bruwier, D. and Cobben, A. (1975) 'La Reduction d'un Comportement Stereotype chez un Enfant arriere Mental Profond: Comparaison de Cinq Methodes', *Schweizerische Zeitschrift fur Psychologie und Ihre Anwendungen Reme Suisse de Psychologie Pure et Applique, 34,* 1–18

Lancioni, G.E., Smeets, P.M., Ceccarani, P.S., Capodaglio, L. and Campanari, G. (1984) 'Effects of Gross Motor Activities on Severe Self-Injurious Tantrums of Multihandicapped Individuals', *Applied Research in Mental Retardation, 5,* 471–82

Leudar, I. and Fraser, W. (1986) 'Behaviour Disturbance and its Assessment' in J. Hogg and N.V. Raynes (eds.), *Assessment in Mental Handicap; A Guide to Tests, Batteries and Checklists,* Croom Helm, London

Lockwood, K. and Bourland, G. (1982) 'Reduction of Self-Injurious Behaviors by Reinforcement and Toy Use', *Mental Retardation, 20,* 169–73

McDaniel, G., Kocim, R. and Barton, L.E. (1984) 'Reducing Self-Stimulatory Mouthing Behaviors in Deaf-Blind Children', *Journal of Visual Impairment and Blindness, 78,* 23–6

Marks, H.E. and Wade, R. (1981) 'A Device for Reducing Object Destruction Among Institutionalised Mentally Retarded Persons', *Mental Retardation, 19,* 181–82

Martin, J., Weller, S. and Matson, J. (1977) 'Eliminating Object-Transferring by a Profoundly Retarded Female by Overcorrection', *Psychological Reports, 40,* 779–82

Murphy, G. (1985) 'Self-Injurious Behaviour in the Mentally Handicapped: An Update', *Association for Child Psychology and Psychiatry Newsletter, 7,* 2–11

Nihira, K. (1978) 'Dimensions of Maladaptive Behavior in Institutionalized Mentally Retarded Persons' in J.D. Swartz, R.K. Eyman, C.C. Cleland and R. O'Grady (eds.), *The Profoundly Mentally Retarded: Fourth Annual Conference Proceedings,* Western Research Conference

Nihira, K., Foster, R., Shellhaas, M. and Leland, H. (1974) *AAMD Adaptive Behavior Scale, 1974 Revision,* American Association on Mental Deficiency, Washington, D.C.

Porterfield, J., Blunden, R. and Blewitt, E. (1980) 'Improving Environments for Profoundly Handicapped Adults', *Behavior Modification, 4,* 225–41

Prescott, J.W. (1976) 'Somatosensory Deprivation and its Relationship to the Blind' in Z.S. Jastrzembska (ed.), *The Effects of Blindness and Other Impairments in Early Development,* American Foundation for the Blind, New York

Reid, J.G., Tombaugh, J.N. and Heuvel, K.V. (1981) 'Application of Contingent Physical Restraint to Suppress Stereotyped Body Rocking of Profoundly Mentally Retarded Persons', *American Journal of Mental Deficiency, 86,* 78–85

Rincover, A. and Devany, J. (1982) 'The Application of Sensory Extinction Procedures to Self-Injury', *Analysis and Intervention in Developmental Disabilities, 2,* 67–81

Schlesinger, H.S. and Meadow, K.P. (1972) *Sound and Sign: Childhood Deafness and Mental Health,* University of California Press, Berkeley

Schroeder, S.R., Mulick, J.A. and Rojahn, J. (1980) 'The Definition, Taxonomy, Epidemiology, and Ecology of Self-Injurious Behavior', *Journal of Autism and Developmental Disorders, 10,* 417–32

Schroeder, S.R., Mulick, J.A. and Schroeder, L.S. (1979) 'Management of Severe Behavior Problems of the Retarded' in N.R. Ellis (ed.), *Handbook of Mental Deficiency Research: Psychological Theory and Research,* 2nd edn. Lawrence Erlbaum, Hillside, N.J.

Silverman, K., Watanabe, K., Marshall, A.M. and Baer, D.M. (1984) 'Reducing Self-Injury and Corresponding Self-Restraint through the Strategic Use of Protective Clothing', *Journal of Applied Behavior Analysis, 17,* 545–52

Singh, N.N., Dawson, M.J. and Manning, P. (1981a) 'Effects of Spaced Responding DRL on the Stereotyped Behavior of Profoundly Retarded Persons', *Journal of Applied Behavior Analysis, 14,* 521–6

Singh, N.N., Dawson, M.J. and Manning, P. (1981b) 'The Effects of Physical Restraint on Self-Injurious Behaviour', *Journal of Mental Deficiency Research, 25,* 207–16

Singh, N.N., Winton, A.S. and Dawson, M.J. (1982) 'Suppression of Antisocial Behavior by Facial Screening Using Multiple Baseline and Alternating Treatment Designs', *Behavior Therapy, 13,* 511–20

Stevens, E.A. (1971) 'Some Effects of Tempo Changes on Stereotyped Rocking Movements of Low-Level Mentally Retarded Subjects', *American Journal of Mental Deficiency, 76,* 76–81

Warren, S.A. and Burns, N.R. (1970) 'Crib Confinement as a Factor in Repetitive and Stereotyped Behavior in Retardates', *Mental Retardation, 8,* 25–8

Wieseler, N.A., Hanson, R.H., Chamberlain, T.P. and Thompson, T. (1985) 'Functional Taxonomy of Stereotypic and Self-Injurious Behavior', *Mental Retardation, 23,* 230–4

Williams, C. (1978) 'Strategies of Intervention with the Profoundly Retarded Visually-Handicapped Child: A Brief Report of a Study of Stereotypy', *Occasional Papers of the British Psychological Society, 2,* 68–72

Williams, J., Schroeder, S.R. and Rojahn, J. (1978) 'Effects of Environmental Enrichment and Contingent Teacher Interaction on the Effectiveness of Time-Out for Self-Injurious Behavior', Paper presented at the Gatlinburg Conference on Mental Retardation, Gatlinburg, Ten.

AUTHOR INDEX

Numbers in italics indicate pages where a full reference is given

SUBJECT INDEX